8138TH ARMY UNIT HOSPITAL TRAINS

KOREAN WAR

KB TAYLOR
www.kb-taylor.com

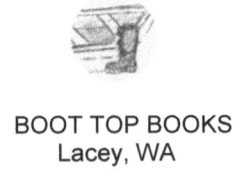

BOOT TOP BOOKS
Lacey, WA

8138th AU Hospital Trains Korean War is a work of nonfiction: letters, articles, and photographs from the Virginia Taylor collection. Included are telephone interviews, correspondence, and photographs from Donald Verstraete.

Copyright© 2021 by Karen Bishop - All Rights Reserved

Library of Congress Cataloging-in-Publication Data
Bishop, Karen (KB Taylor)

LCCN: 2021940241

8138th AU Hospital Trains Korean War/KB Taylor-1st ed.
p. cm: includes bibliographical references.
Summary: Based on the collections of Virginia M. Taylor and Don Verstraete

ISBN: 9781733369756

1. 8138th Hospital Trains Korea. 2. Hospital Trains Korea. 3.) Wartime Medical Transport. 4. Nurses and Medics of the Korean War. (Revision 2 update, pg 51 Dr. Hukill)

Front Cover: 1st Lt. Virginia Taylor and Crew Chief Andy Anderson caring for a wounded Greek soldier.
Back Cover: Train #105 kitchen car. Nurse 1st Lt. Virginia Taylor red curtains for the Kitchen/Dining car. 8138th AU Hospital Train #105.

Printed in the United States of America
June 2021
Boot Top Books
Lacey, WA

10 9 8 7 6 5 4 3 2

AUTHOR'S NOTE

Receipt of my aunt Virginia Taylor's Korean War scrapbook of 200+ personal photos, news articles, and letters written to family, spurred me to do further research on the **8138th AU Hospital Trains**.

Requests all hauntingly the same: *Would like to hear from anyone who remembers the trains; we did a good job; unit never got much mention in the news; the unit seems to have dropped off the face of the earth.*

After researching websites, ancestry sites, and obituaries, I wrote twenty-five letters. To my delight, I received a reply from medic Don Verstraete. Don had served on the 8138th Hospital Train #106 from April 1952 through May 1953.

Don's train service in Korea intertwined with my aunt's, however, the two never met. Another crossing of paths was in 1949 at Fort Sam Houston, San Antonio, Texas. Don received his medical training during the same period that Virginia Taylor was stationed there completing hers.

Over the past two years, Don and I have corresponded through e-mails, letters, and telephone conversations. Virginia's letters and photos, and Don's first-hand accounts capture the importance of the hospital trains during the Korean War.

On August 20, 1952, the 8138th Unit received a Presidential Citation. Don and Virginia were both there. Virginia stated the following in a letter:

> *TOMORROW at 1300 the hospital train unit is being presented with a Presidential Unit Citation down at the pier. We all have to stand formation—8 nurses, 6 doctors, 120 corpsman, and 25 men from the maintenance section will get the award. We all think it's pretty wonderful.*

I agree! And justly deserved.
Author – KB Taylor

June 1950, Army Corps Nurse Virginia Taylor arrived in the Far East one week after her twenty-third birthday and several weeks before the start of the Korean War. First stationed at Ryukyus Hospital, Okinawa, Japan, she was 500 miles from the frontlines and a two-hour plane ride away. The effects of the war were felt daily through troop movements, blackouts and sirens, and the arrival of wounded from the frontlines.

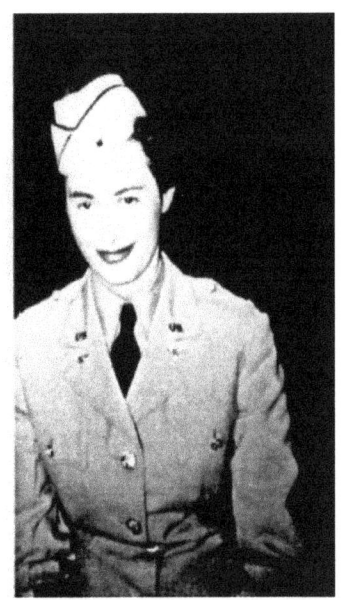

(Photos courtesy of Virginia Taylor collection)

Okinawa, July 3, 1950 Excerpts of Virginia Taylor's letter to her parents:

Last week we all had a typhoon alert. The typhoon "Elsie" ripped up an island 75 miles below us but missed Okinawa except for the winds of 50 miles per hour. Last week we also got this Korea alert so things are really cooking. This little strip of island is the "Powder Keg of the Pacific" and I will say, I'm not too happy about sitting here right now. Okinawa is like a Giant Stationary Aircraft Carrier, having eight large air bases big enough to land B-36's. Of course, it has an impenetrable radar screen and AAA guns and tanks and hundreds of infantry riflemen swarming everywhere, so at least we are ready.

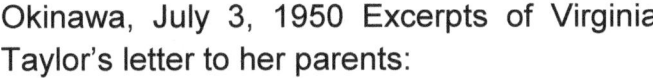

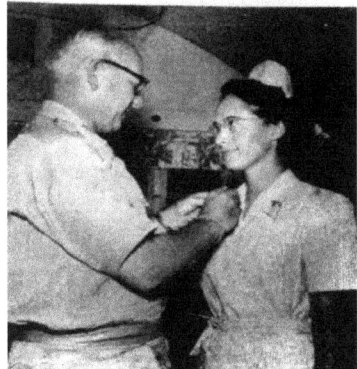

Lt. Virginia M. Taylor, Rycom Army hospital is shown just as she changed from Second Lt. to First Lt. Colonel Walter H. Stevenson, commanding officer of the 8114th Service Detachment, pinned on her new bars.

UNITED STATES AIR FORCE
Okinawa

July 3 1950
Monday
0815

Dearest Folks,

Haven't heard but one time since I've been here from you so don't know whether you're on your way North or just whats cooking - but I figured I'd better be a writting anyway and I guess it'll be there when you get back. I sent my last letter to you all to Rosie.

Well, Okinawa has finally quit raining and the days are a little hot but one could not ask for anything as beautiful as the Sun rise and Sun set on the China Sea. As I stated previously the Hospital is built on the Beach of the China Sea which gives us a cool breeze all Day and night.

We work a 5 day week and I guess I shouldn't really use the term "work" - cause we don't do any compared to what I've been used to.

Last week we all had a typhoon alert. The typhoon "Elsie" ripped up an Island 75 miles below us but missed Okinawa except for winds of 50 miles per hour. Last week we also got this Korea alert so things are really cooking. This little strip of Island is the Powder Keg of the Pacific and I will say, I'm not to happy about sitting here right now. Okinawa is like a Giant, Stationary air craft carrier. Having 18 large air bases big enough to land B-36's - Of course it has an impenatrable Radar Screen and AAA Guns and Tanks and Hundreds of Infantry rifle men swarming everywhere so at least we are ready.

Last evening 6 of us girls rode down to White Beach, on the Pacific side and watched a huge

August 25, 1951 Excerpts of Virginia Taylor letter to her parents:

With this letter I close the chapter of my life on little Okinawa Shimco. Come take off time on Thursday, Captain McDonald, Lt. Hardesty, Captain Nichols, Lt. Arnold and myself will head north. We have been chosen for "Chosin." We are not sure yet of our assignments. We report to Taegu, Korea. <u>I am going to ask for the Hospital Train which carries wounded from Seoul to Pusan.</u> I am welcoming a change – and am looking forward to new faces and places, as are the others. This tour of duty will put me 6 months closer to home. I guess it's like jumping out of the frying pan into the fire, but it will be good experience and someone has to do the job.

My room's a mess – we can only take a duffle bag with us and it's so hard to choose what we will need most. Our footlockers will be stored in Japan until our 6-month tour is finished. One thing, it'll be good to see snow again this winter after all this heat.

```
                HEADQUARTERS
           EIGHTH UNITED STATES ARMY KOREA (EUSAK)
                Office of the Commanding General
                        APO 301

SPECIAL ORDERS                                    17 December 1951
NUMBER   351                EXTRACT                          RMK

     3.  Fol changes in asg directed. DD Form 415 reflecting address of orgn
to which trf will be furnished unit mail clerk. WP. PCS. EDCSA 22 Dec 51.
TDN. TBGAA. TBMAA. Tvl by rail auth.

                              REL SG              ASG

1STLT CORINNE S BRYANT     21st Evac Hosp APO 301   Mbl A Surg Hosp 8209th
        ANC 3449 (Cau)                                  AU APO 301
1STLT ROSEMARY F MAHONEY          do                        do
        ANC 3449 (Cau)
1STLT SARA L ABLES                do              22d Evac Hosp APO 301
        ANC 3437 (Cau)
1STLT VIRGINIA M TAYLOR           do              Hosp Train 8138th AU
        ANC 3449 (Cau)                                  APO 301
```

December 17, 1951 Orders permanently assigning Virginia Taylor to the 8138th AU Hospital Train. (She had already been working the trains since SEPTEMBER 1951.)

L to R: Virginia Taylor, Sara Ables, Corinne Byrant, Rosemary Mahoney. All 1st Lts and nurses at the 21st EVAC Hospital, Pusan. Their re-assignments are listed above.

January 1949, nineteen-year-old Don Verstraete enlisted into the U.S. Army. After eight weeks of basic training in Breckenridge, Kentucky, he headed to San Antonio, Texas for Field Medical School training.

July 1949 – Sept 1951, he was stationed in Germany at the 97th General Hospital. First, as a corpsman, and then promoted to a Hospital Ward Master. Before shipping out to the Far East, he was dispatched to the States (Indiana) for six months.

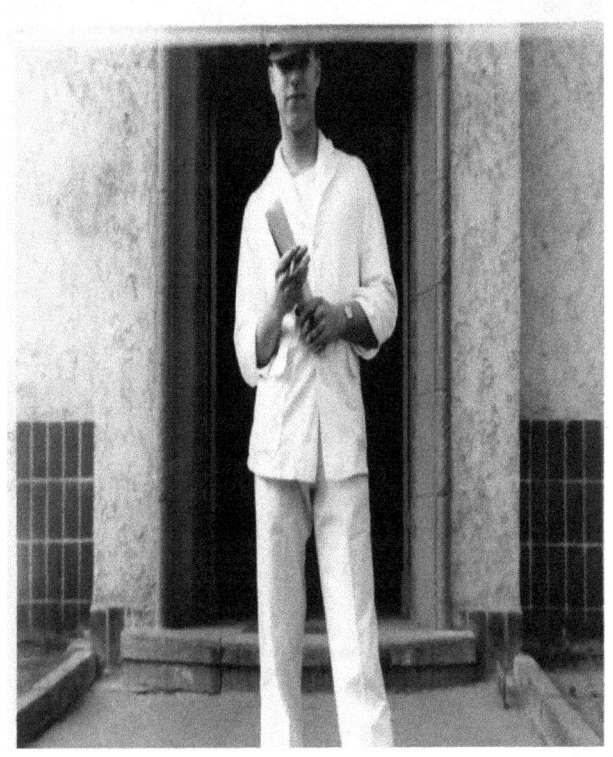

20-year-old Don Verstraete in Germany
(Photo courtesy of Don Verstraete collection)

March 1952, twenty-two-year-old Don arrived in Tokyo, Japan. A week later, he transferred to Korea and assigned to the 421 Medical Collecting Company as a Medic on the 8138th Army Unit Hospital Trains. From April 1952 to May 1953, he lived aboard Hospital Train #106 and served as a car commander. He also participated in the first Operation Little Switch POW Exchange on April 20, 1953.

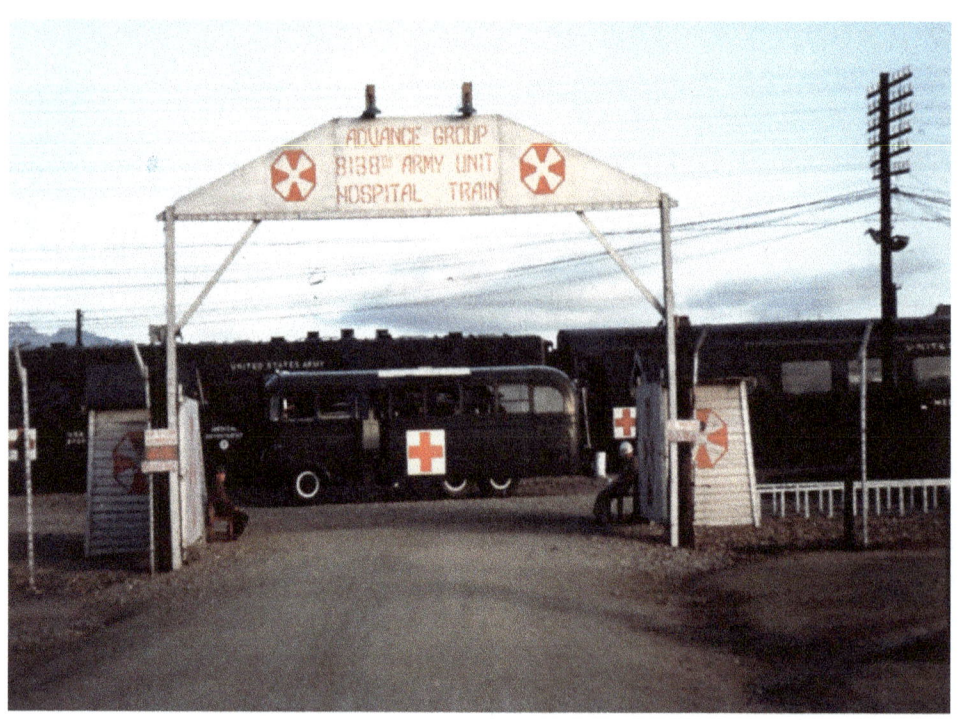

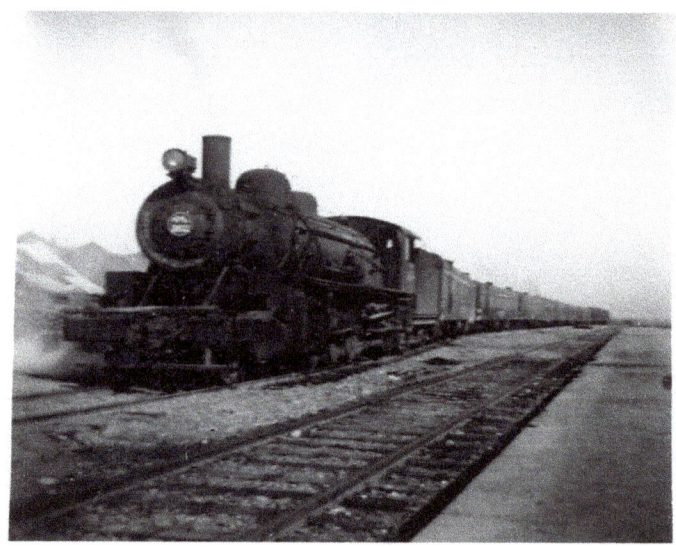

8138th AU Hospital Train #105

(Photos courtesy of Virginia Taylor collection)

THE KOREAN WAR OVERVIEW
(1950-1953)

After years of turmoil between China, Japan, and Russia to overtake Korea, the Russo-Japanese War of 1904 put Korea under Japanese rule. Japan ousted the Korean emperor, created a colonial regime, and annexed Korea in 1910. It wasn't until 1945 when Japan surrendered to the Allies ending WWII, that Korea's fate was redefined again. The United States, Great Britain, Russia, and China agreed that the Japanese troops above the 38th parallel would surrender to the Soviets and the troops south of the line to the American forces. The United States considered the divide temporary, but it soon became clear that the Soviets regarded it as permanent.

The United Nations sought for unification of Korea, but the Soviet Union refused and created a communist regime under the leadership of Kim Il-Sung. In 1948, South Korea formed the Republic of Korea (ROK) and elected Syngman Rhee as its first president by National Assembly.

Border skirmishes erupted between the two sides, each ruler wanting all of Korea under their control. The Soviet-backed North Korean regime continued to build up its army, and on June 25, 1950, invaded the South.

The U.N. Security Council demanded immediate cessation of hostilities and withdrawal of North Korean forces to the 38th parallel.[1] President Truman relayed orders to General Douglas MacArthur at the Far East Command in Tokyo. He also ordered the Seventh Fleet from its current location in Philippine and Ryukyu waters to Japan. Later, he redirected the bulk of the fleet to Taiwan.

North Korea ignored the U.N. demands, which forced the U.N. Security Council, on June 27, 1950, to notify the member nations to furnish military assistance to South Korea. *This was the first time since the United Nations founding that it reacted to aggression with a decision to use armed force.*[2]

On June 30, 1950, President Truman broadened the range of U.S. air and naval support and authorized General MacArthur to use all of the Eighth U.S. Army ground forces stationed in Japan and the 28th Regimental

Combat Team on Okinawa. None of these units were battle ready and were underpowered.

The first troops from the United States landed in Korea on July 1, 1950. Australia's 77th Fighter Squadron was the first foreign unit to arrive in Korea on July 2, 1950. It attached to the 35th U.S. Fighter Group.[3] Ground, air, and naval forces represented by twenty U.N. Members and one nonmember nation, arrived in phases, but it was the United States that provided most of the weapons, equipment, and logistical support.[4]

President Truman never asked Congress to pass an official declaration of war and declared the Korean War a "police action." A unified command in the field was designated the United Nations Command (UNC) and put under the leadership of General MacArthur.

By the fall of 1950, the U.S. altered its objective from containment of North Korea to liberation from Communist rule. This resulted in the People's Republic of China to intervene and created an entirely new war.[5] During the winter of 1950-1951 and through the summer of 1951, the conflict shifted from a dangerous struggle to one that could have expanded into a global war.[6]

November 1950 was one of the most horrific of the battles. As the American and South Korean forces drove the North Koreans back to their border, several hundred thousand Chinese troops amassed around the Chosin *(Changjin)* Reservoir. The Allies, caught by surprise, were outnumbered six to one. This battle was fought over some of the roughest terrain and harshest winters of the war. A Siberian cold front had plunged temperatures to as low as -36 degrees. Medical supplies and blood plasma froze. Tending to wounds risked gangrene and frostbite. Batteries for Jeeps and radios malfunctioned. Lubrication in the guns gelled. Springs in firing pins would not strike hard enough to fire or would jam.[7]

Over the course of this war (1950-1953), one million seven-hundred eighty-nine thousand military personnel served from the United States (91.5%) and one-hundred and sixty-six thousand from fifteen other countries (8.5%).

Estimated Foreign Military Personnel who served in Korea 1950-1953[8]

Country	Total	% Total	Arrival Date
Australia	17,164	10.34%	Jul-50
Belgium	3,498	2.11%	Jan-51
Canada	27,000	16.27%	Jul-50
Columbia	6,200	3.73%	Jun-51
Ethiopia	3,518	2.12%	May-51
France	4,000	2.41%	Jul-50
Greece	5,000	3.01%	Dec-50
Luxembourg	89	0.054%	Jan-51
Netherlands	5,300	3.19%	Nov-50
New Zealand	4,500	2.71%	Aug-50
Philippines	7,420	4.47%	Sep-50
South Africa	811	0.49%	Nov-50
Thailand	6,500	3.92%	Nov-50
Turkey	15,000	9.04%	Oct-50
United Kingdom	60,000	36.14%	Jun-50
TOTAL FOREIGN w/o United States	**166,000**	**100.00%**	

Country	Total	% Total	Arrival Date
FOREIGN (Above)	166,000	8.5%	
UNITED STATES [9]	1,789,000	91.5%	Jun-50

Five non-combatant nations provided hospital personnel and medical units: India, Sweden, Norway, Denmark and Italy (the Non-United Nations country). Hundreds served from these countries during the war.

Department of Veterans Affairs/America's Wars[10]	KOREAN WAR 1950-1953
U.S. Service members (worldwide)	5,720,000
Total serving (in theater- Korea)	**1,789,000**

In theater: Served in Korea during the war 1950-1953. Non-theater: those who were stationed in the United States, Germany, and other offsite posts. NOT Korea. (Civilian lost for both North and South Korea has been estimated in the millions.)

Estimated Foreign Military Personnel Casualties in the Korean War 1950-1953[11]

Country	Killed	Wounded	Missing	Killed	Wounded	Missing
Australia	339	1216	72	8.6%	10.1%	4.0%
Belgium	101	336	5	2.6%	2.8%	0.3%
Canada	516	1,212	32	13.1%	10.0%	1.8%
Columbia	163	448	28	4.1%	3.7%	1.6%
Ethiopia	121	536	0	3.1%	4.4%	0.0%
France	262	1,008	19	6.6%	8.4%	1.1%
Greece	192	543	2	4.9%	4.5%	0.1%
Luxembourg	2	13	0	0.1%	0.1%	0.0%
Netherlands	120	645	3	3.0%	5.3%	0.2%
New Zealand	23	79	1	0.6%	0.7%	0.1%
Philippines	122	299	57	3.1%	2.5%	3.2%
South Africa	34	0	8	0.9%	0.0%	0.4%
Thailand	129	1,139	5	3.3%	9.4%	0.3%
Turkey	741	2,068	407	18.8%	17.1%	22.7%
United Kingdom	1,078	2,674	1060	27.3%	21.0%	64.4%
TOTAL FOREIGN w/o USA	**3,943**	**12,075**	**1,796**	**100.0%**	**100.0%**	**100.0%**
Foreign (Above)	3,943	12,075	1,796	9.7%	10.5%	18.0%
United States	36,574	103,284	8,176	90.3%	89.5%	82.0%
GRAND TOTAL	40,517	115,359	9,972	100.0%	100.0%	100.0%

Total Casualties [12]

SOUTH KOREA	843,572 – 988,400
NORTH KOREA	520,000 – 900,000
CHINA	900,000
SOVIET UNION	299

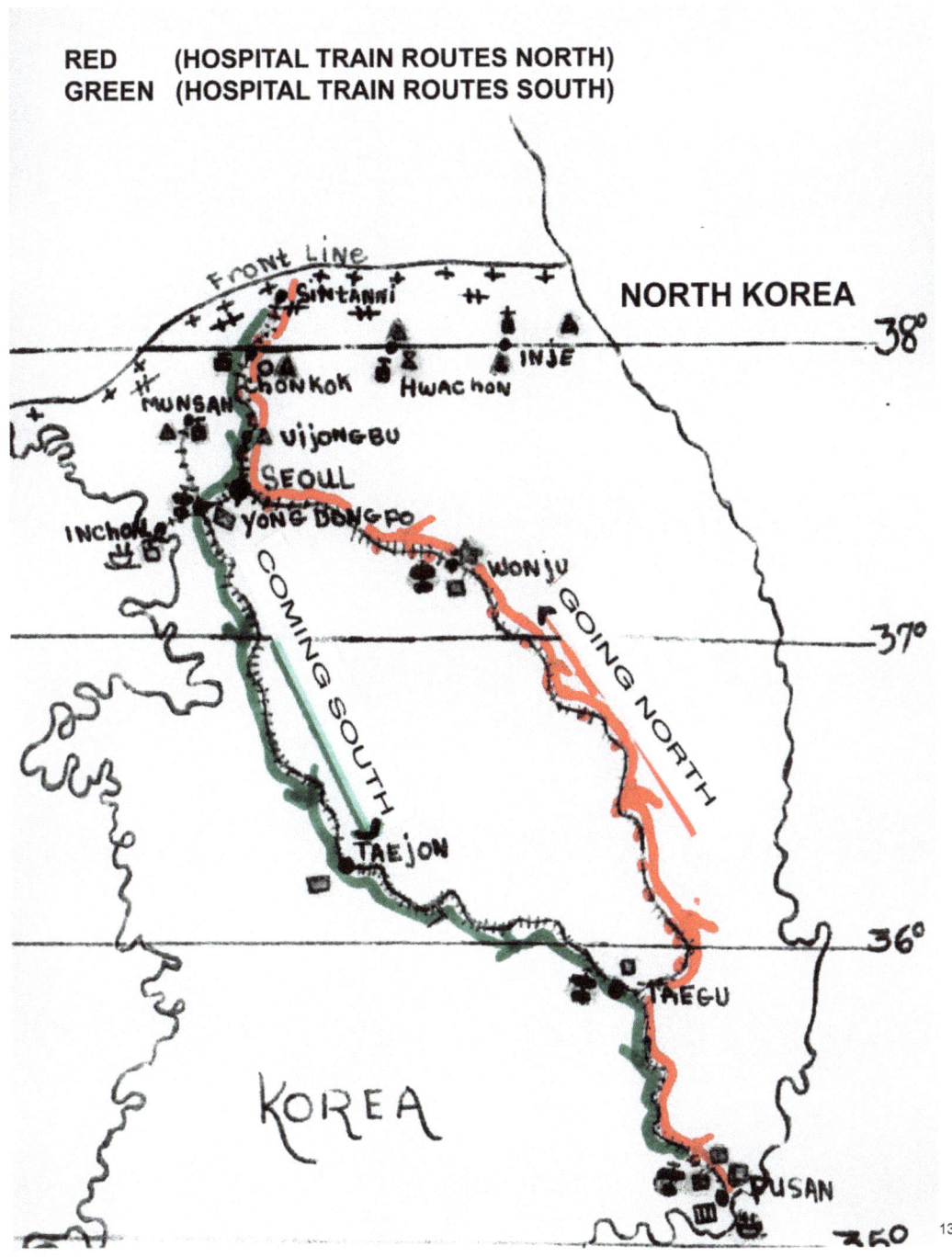

JUNE 25, 1950   North Korea invaded South Korea
JUNE 27, 1950   President Truman ordered U.S. Forces to Korea
JUNE 27, 1950   U.N. Security Council notified member nations for support
JULY 01, 1950   The first U.S. troops from the States arrived to Korea

At the start of the Korean War, there were no hospital trains and very few hospitals. Nurses from the field and evacuation hospitals accompanied patients on converted Korean trains and rotated on litters. <u>Patients had to be loaded through the windows</u>, but those with long leg casts or splints presented a problem. To meet this emergency, the window was removed and the foot left protruding through the opening.[14]

> *"That wasn't so bad," one nurse said. "It was hot and we needed the extra circulation of air, but the railroad went through so many tunnels and there was so much soot and cinder that we had to cover our patient's faces with damp clothes to protect them."* [15]

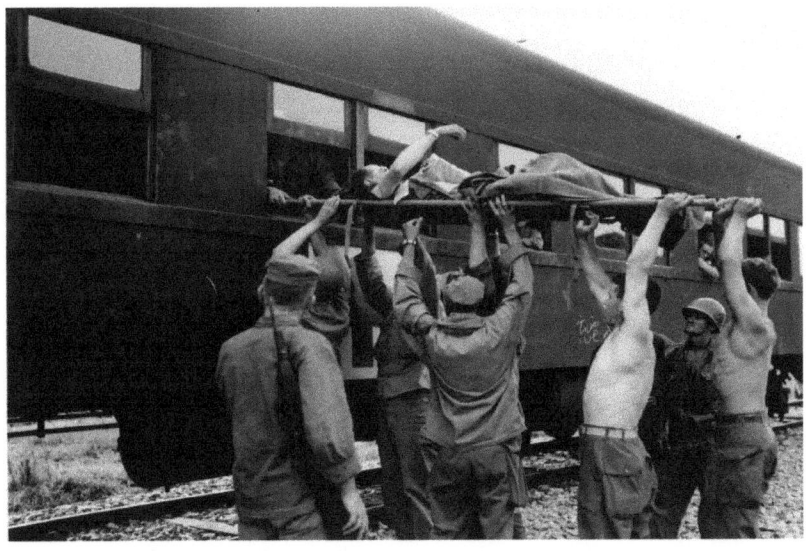

(Photo courtesy of Virginia Taylor collection) [16]

August 1, 1950, the Army's surgeon general received a request from General MacArthur for two hospital trains for use in the Far East. By year-end, two ten-car trains formed a continuous shuttle between the front and Pusan.[17]

Between November 1950 and March 1951, sixty-two hospital-ward cars, including seven kitchen cars, arrived in Korea. All shipped from the United States and constructed in 1944 and 1945 for stateside service. The standard train consisted of thirteen cars: eight ward cars, a kitchen, dining, and pharmacy car, an officer/personnel car, two orderly cars, and one utility car.[18]

By the end of 1951, hospital trains #20 and #22 had combined into one unit: the **8138th Army Unit Hospital Trains**.[19] With the formation of the new unit, the cars were divided into EIGHT hospital trains. (Train #101 through #108.) Each train had seven cars: six hospital-ward cars and one kitchen, dining, and pharmacy car.[20] The kitchen cars were converted from baggage cars and self-contained with hot and cold water, electrical, and a coal-fired stove and oven.

All eight trains headquartered on the Pier 1 dock, in Pusan Harbor, Korea with continuous runs to the front. As one train headed north, another returned with wounded.[21]

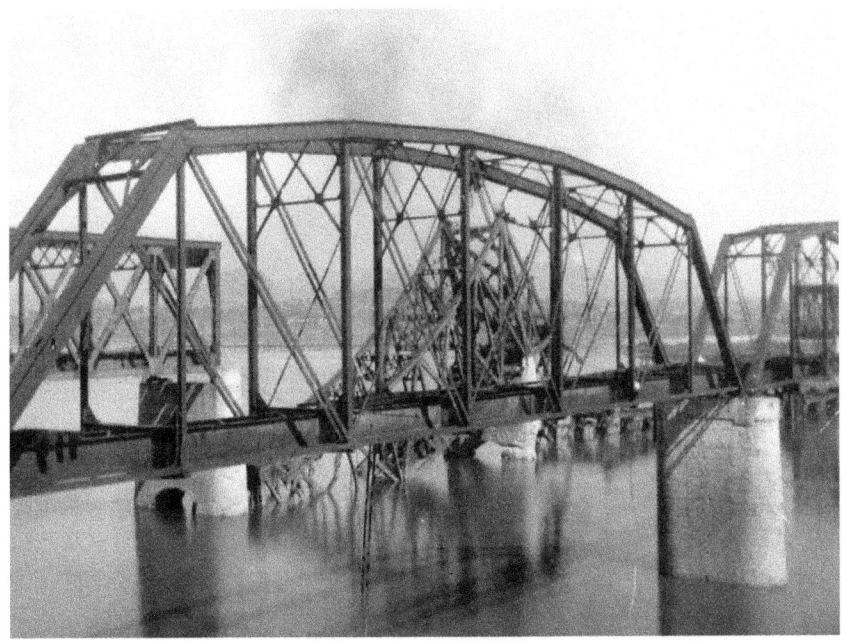

Han River Bridge reconstructed by Army Engineers
(Bombed bridge behind)

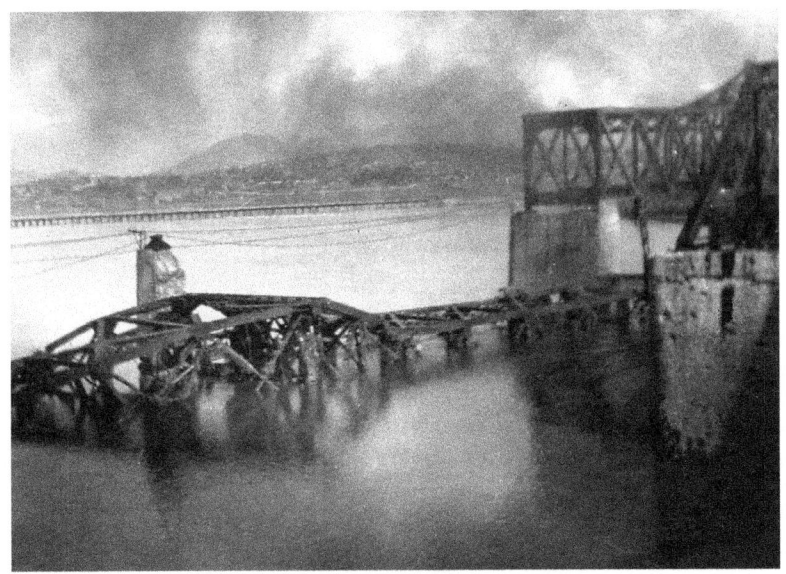

Bombed bridge over the Han River

(Photos courtesy of Virginia Taylor collection)

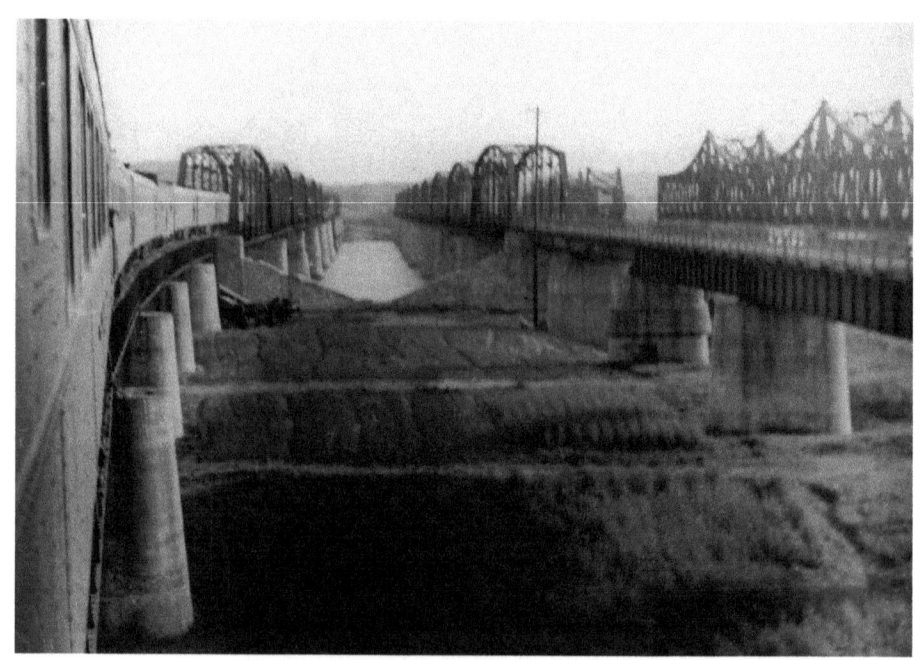

Hospital Train 106 crossing reconstructed bridge over the
Han River
(Photo courtesy of Don Verstraete collection)

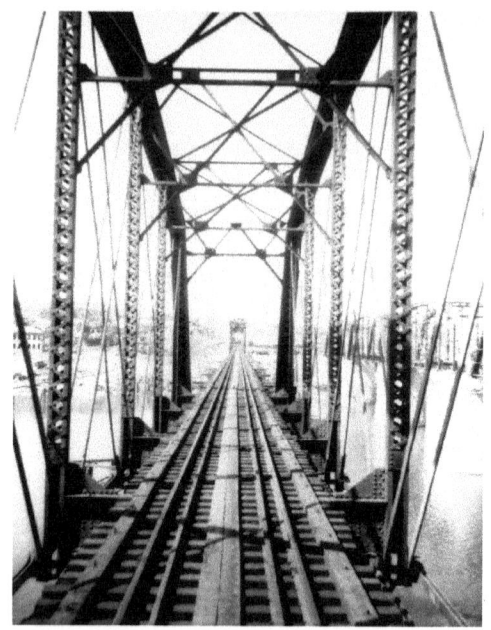

Reconstructed bridge over the Han River
(Photo courtesy Virginia Taylor collection)

TMRS
3rd Transportation Military Railway Service

The TMRS played a vital role in the Korean War. The perseverance and bravery of the railroad battalions aided in the building, repair, and maintenance of tracks, tunnels, railway facilities, and blown-up bridges. Locomotives and water pumps along the lines required constant maintenance and the Korean equipment, smaller and badly worn, had to be retrofit and fixed. The tortuous mountainous tracks had rotten ties, loose spikes, and non-existent tie plates plus 300 tunnels and 1000 bridges in need of maintenance or repair.[22]

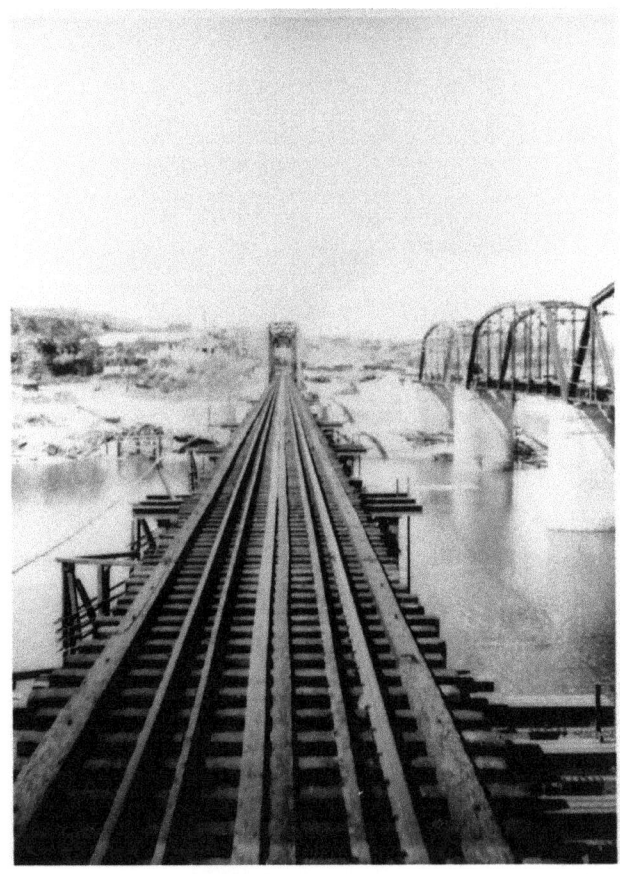

Reconstructed bridge
(Photo courtesy of Virginia Taylor collection)

Prior to the Korean War, the vast majority of the Korean National Railroad (KNR) had been built, maintained, and operated by the Japanese from 1905-1945 (including what would become North Korea.) [23]

Due to a shortage of motor vehicles and poor road conditions, the EUSA (Eighth United States Army) and Republic of Korea Army depended heavily on the KNR for overland transportation.[24] The immense traffic demands and inexperience of the management and crews overwhelmed the KNR, making it impossible to handle the burden. In July 1950, EUSA negotiated the transfer of operation control from the ROK (Republic of Korea) government to the U.S. Army.

July 1950, the 8059th Army Unit arrived in Pusan and assumed supervision of all railroad operations and maintenance while the KNR oversaw the locomotive crew. The 709th Transportation Railway Grand Division controlled operations and movements of the KNR while establishing communication post along the rails. As additional battalions joined the initial set up, Korean personnel were crucial as well.

On August 26, 1950, the **3rd Transportation Military Railway Service (TMRS)** at Pusan was formed. The 8059th Army Unit and 709th Transportation Railway Grand Division were inactivated. Their assets were transferred to the **3rd** TMRS 714th Battalion and 765th Railway Shop Battalion. During this period, bands of North Korean guerillas added danger and difficulties of rail transportation. The 714th Battalion more than once engaged in combat, even though combat was not their primary task.[25]

July 1951, the TMRS 714th Battalion left Korea and was replaced by two units: the 712th and 724th Transportation Railway Operating Battalions (TROB). The 712th TROB, headquartered at Yongdongpo, handled all rail traffic north of Taejon. The 724th TROB, headquartered at Pusan, handled rail traffic from Pusan to Taejon. The 765th Transportation Railway Shop Battalion (TRSB) remained and was stationed at Pusan.

3rd TMRS Runs Busy Railroad
Express, Flyer Carry Burden of Korean Travel

WITH 3rd TMRS—Everyone wants to travel in Korea. In fact, nearly everyone must travel at one time or another over facilities of the 3rd Transportation Military Railway Service.

Although air travel is a big factor, the average foot soldier of the United Nations Command finds himself in a busy passenger terminal, getting his orders processed so that he can travel on the EUSAK Express or Flyer, trains operating between Seoul and Pusan.

If he is a part of a large troop movement, replacement coaches will be made available at a railhead.

TRAVEL ON the EUSAK Express or Flyer, northbound or southbound, is not limited to military personnel. Civilians employed by the United Nations or the American embassy, often board one of the trains.

President and Mrs. Syngman Rhee sometimes climb on their private railroad car for a trip from the provisional capital in Pusan to the gutted capital city of Seoul.

Occasionally, a woman, perhaps a wife of a missionary or a Red Cross employee, or an embassy official, arrives for a trip, usually clad in fatigue clothing, but nevertheless, relieving the drab OD monotony of hundreds of soldiers.

THE TURKS, Belgians, and French arrive with their small rakish berets and colorful national and unit designations: the Australians with their big slouch hats; the Greeks board the train, replete with luxurious mustaches.

They are all going somewhere. Some are reporting to a replacement depot for rotation home, some are returning from R&R in Japan; some are returning from the frontlines, and some are traveling in connection with UN agency activities.

Now and then in the dark a crowded troop train will pass by headed north, or <u>a silent hospital train will glide by.</u>

This is one of the most united of all the United Nations activities in Korea, and is an interesting, colorful activity.

3d TMRS Runs Busy Railroad

Express, Flyer Carry Burden Of Korean Travel

WITH 3D TMRS—Everyone wants to travel in Korea. In fact, nearly everyone must travel at one time or another over facilities of the 3d Transportation Military Railway Service.

Although air travel is a big factor, the average foot soldier of the United Nations Command finds himself in a busy passenger terminal, getting his orders processed so that he can travel on the EUSAK Express or Flyer, trains operating between Seoul and Pusan.

If he is a part of a large troop movement, replacement coaches will be made available at a railhead.

TRAVEL ON the EUSAK Express or Flyer, northbound or southbound, is not limited to military personnel. Civilians employed by the United Nations or the American embassy, often board one of the trains.

President and Mrs. Syngman Rhee sometimes climb on their private railroad car for a trip from the provisional capital in Pusan to the gutted capital city of Seoul.

Occasionally, a woman, perhaps the wife of a missionary, or a Red Cross employe, or an embassy official, arrives for a trip, usually clad in fatigue clothing, but nevertheless relieving the drab OD monotony of hundreds of soldiers.

THE TURKS, Belgians, and French, arrive with their small, rakish berets and colorful national and unit designations; the Australians with their big slouch hats; the Greeks board the train, replete with luxurious mustaches.

They are all going somewhere. Some are reporting to a replacement depot for rotation home; some are returning from R&R in Japan; some are returning from the frontlines, and some are traveling in connection with UN agency activities.

Now and then in the dark a crowded troop train will pass by, headed north, or a silent hospital train will glide by.

This is one of the most united of all the United Nations activities in Korea, and is an interesting, colorful activity.

"TRANS-MEDICS"

TO A CAUSALTY direct from the front, nothing is more reassuring than to be taken in hand by personnel of the "Trans-Medics" Hospital Train Evacuation Service.

The medical half of the Mercy Train partnership is composed of nine Army doctors, nine specially trained Army nurses, and 220 enlisted medical technicians—all members of the 8138th Army Unit Hospital Trains. The 3rd Transportation Military Railway Service provides the rolling wards, kitchens and dining cars as their contribution to the life saving team.

For the 60 Stateside-constructed, hospital-pullman ward cars, the 3rd TMRS maintains a ratio of one-to-ten kitchen and dining cars. In addition to these hospital trains, the men of the TC maintain and operate four bus-trains. These unique vehicles are Army ambulance-busses adapted to use either on rails or the Korean dirt trails.

Both steam and diesel locomotives are on call to power the conventional trains. But as the long, cold Asiatic winter approaches, the medics specify that the steam locomotives be used as all cars are steam heated. Even the special PW car, attached to each train to evacuate wounded prisoners, provides maximum comfort under the existing conditions.

The medical staff of individual trains is made up of one doctor and one nurse, plus an enlisted technician per car. The doctor, in addition to his duties as surgeon, is train commander.

But things weren't always this refined in the evacuation of UN wounded in Korea. Until the first mercy train arrived in September 1950, Korean passenger cars were used as hospital cars. Litters were balanced over the seats and heat and sanitary facilities were catch-as-catch-can. Since the arrival of the first train, over 150,000 wounded, including POWs, have been evacuated from the danger of the combat zone.

"TRANS-MEDICS"
(Continued)

Doing maintenance for the hospital trains is the 765th Transportation Railway Shop Battalion. It was in this shop that the hospital train-busses were improved upon so that by a mere four hours of labor, the life-span of their wheel-set was quadrupled. <u>By a flick of a switch, the bus can be changed to a track-bound vehicle or given the freedom of the roads.</u>

On the lighter side are the difficulties sometimes experienced because of a language barrier existing between the medics and some of their patients. One nurse mastered the required phrases needed to converse with the Chinese PWs, but was stymied by the wounded UN Ethiopian soldier. Conversation, necessary before treatment could be given, seemed impossible—then the nurse, remembering the World War II Axis, tried Italian and it worked.

The "Trans-Medics" leave no problem unsolved.

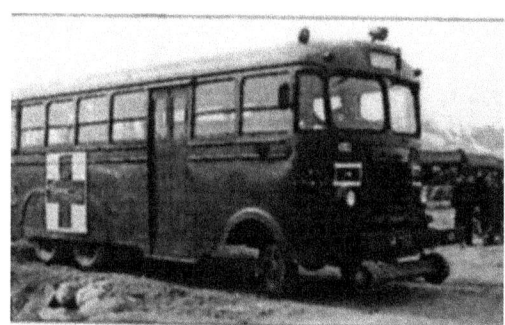

Ambulance hospital bus changed to a track-bound vehicle with a flick of a switch. (Courtesy of National Archives, Signal Corps)

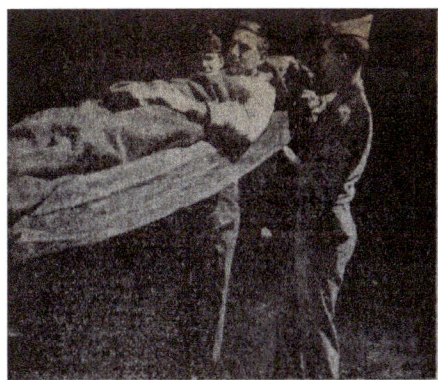

"TRANS-MEDICS" HANDLE LITTER PATIENTS with care. Picked up just a few miles behind the frontlines, this patient is off-loaded from the Mercy Train for further evacuation to a modern hospital.

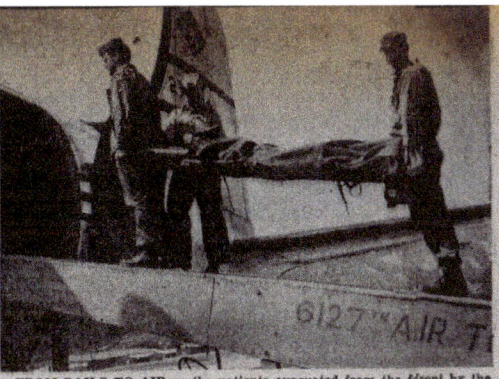

FROM RAILS TO AIR go the patients evacuated from the front by the "Trans-Medics." Flight nurse, Lt. Mary J. Kitterage, checks the records of a litter patient brought to the air terminal by the Mercy Train.

"TRANS-MEDICS"

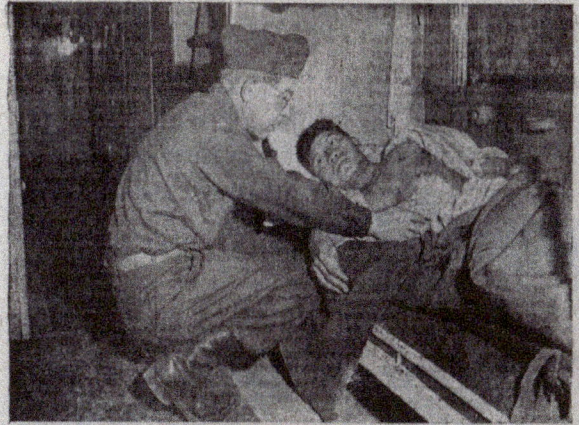

EXPERT MEDICAL ATTENTION is given all patients aboard the evacuation trains. Above, Capt. Gerhard J. Newerla, train commander and surgeon, inspects the wound dressing of Pvt. Willard West of the U.S. 45th Division. Each train is staffed by an Army doctor, nurse, and an enlisted technician per car. (U.S. Army photos by Feinstein)

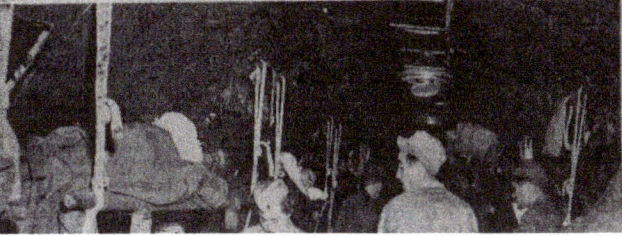

To A CASUALTY direct from the front, nothing is more reassuring than to be taken in hand by personnel of the "Trans-Medics" Hospital Train Evacuation Service.

The medical half of the Mercy Train partnership is composed of nine Army doctors, nine specially trained Army nurses, and 220 enlisted medical technicians—all members of the 8138th Army Unit. The 3d Transportation Military Railway Service provides the rolling wards, kitchens, and dining cars as their contribution to the life saving team.

For the 60 Stateside-constructed, hospital-pullman ward cars, the 3d TMRS maintains a ratio of one-to-ten kitchen and dining cars. In addition to these hospital trains, the men of the TC maintain and operate four bus-trains. These unique vehicles are Army ambulance-busses adapted to use either on rails or the Korean dirt trails.

Both steam and diesel locomotives are on call to power the conventional trains. But as the long, cold Asiatic winter approaches, the medics specify that the steam locomotives be used as all cars are steam heated. Even the special PW car, attached to each train to evacuate wounded prisoners, provides maximum comfort under the existing conditions.

The medical staff of individual trains is made up of one doctor and one nurse, plus an enlisted technician per car. The doctor, in addition to his duties as surgeon, is train commander.

But things weren't always this refined in the evacuation of UN wounded in Korea. Until the first mercy train arrived in September, 1950, Korean passenger cars were used as hospital cars. Litters were balanced over the seats and heat and sanitary facilities were catch-as-catch-can. Since the arrival of the first train, over 150,000 wounded, including PWs, have been evacuated from the danger of the combat zone.

Doing maintenance for the hospital trains is the 765th Transportation Railway Shop Battalion. It was in this shop that the hospital train-busses were improved upon so that by a mere four hours of labor, the life-span of their wheel-set was quadrupled. By a flick of a switch the bus can be changed to a track-bound vehicle or given the free-

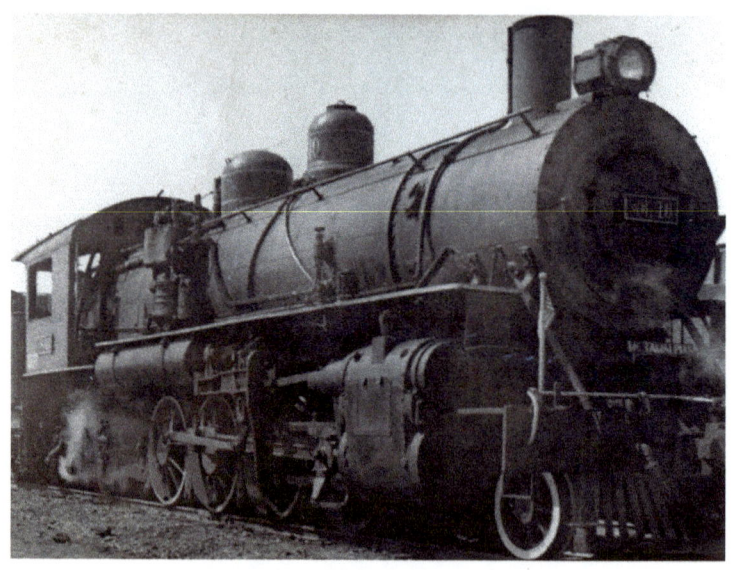

STEAM LOCOMOTIVE (TRAIN 106)
(Photo courtesy of Don Verstraete collection)

(During the cold Asiatic winters, steam locomotives pulled the hospital trains and heated all the cars with steam from their engine.)

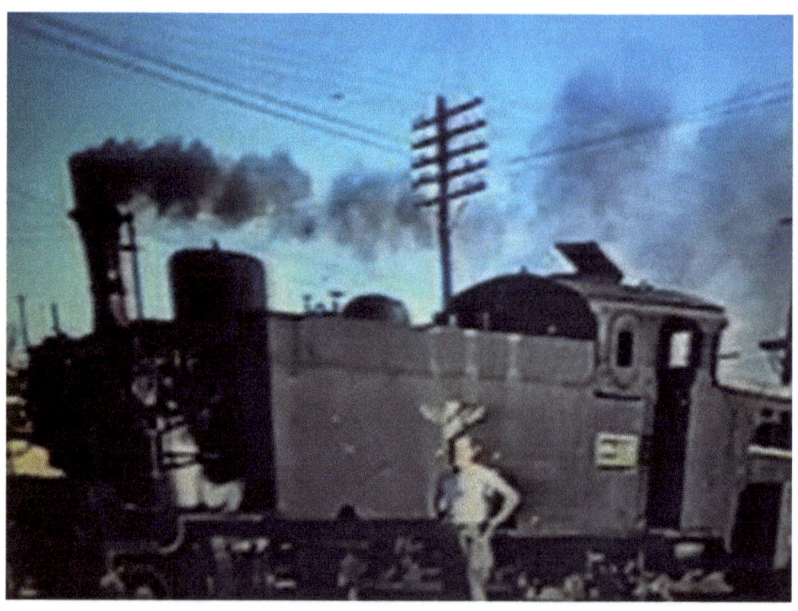

DIESEL LOCOMOTIVE (with smoke) USED IN SUMMER
(Photo courtesy of Virginia Taylor collection)

MEDICAL AIRLIFT OUT of Korea was dependent on good weather. The nearest airfield to the front along the Nakdong River was the K-2 Airfield near Taegu. Due to rough roads and lack of railheads at the airfield, EUSA (Eighth United States Army) preferred to move its casualties by hospital trains to Pusan.[28]

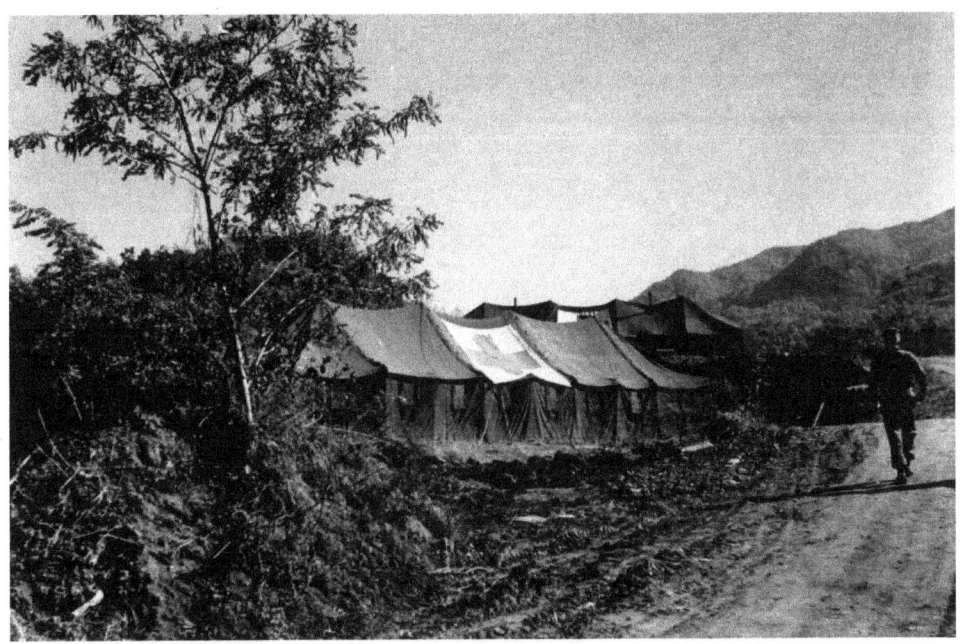

Hospital trains could evacuate casualties directly from the frontline

SINTANNI 2nd Div Collecting Station, North Korea

8,000 yards from enemy lines[29]
(Photo courtesy of Virginia Taylor collection)

Hospital trains began operating from forward railheads in the combat zone to hospitals in Taejon, Taegu, and Pusan. At the Sintanni Collecting Station, wounded were carried to the hospital train on litters. Twenty miles south at the Chonkok Clearing Station many of the wounded arrived by ambulance convoys from nearby MASH units.[30]

The railroad line first extended north from Seoul to Uijonbu, and later to Chorwon, providing a superior supply and evacuation system. Along this line, EUSA placed all forward medical installations, including the all-important MASH units. Critically wounded men were flown by helicopter from battalion aid stations at the front to the nearest MASH hospital.[31]

Often head, chest, and abdominal cases were on an operating table within minutes of being wounded. After their surgeries, a hospital train fully equipped and staffed further evacuated patients to hospitals in the rear.[32]

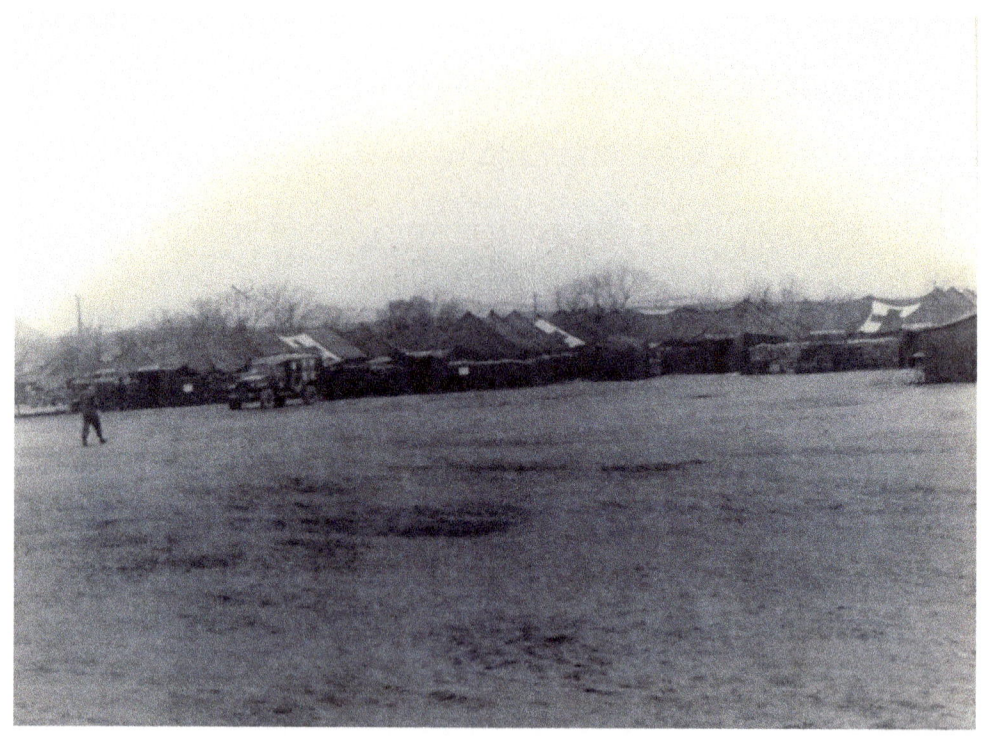

8055 MASH—Four miles from the CHONKOK CLEARING STATION. Patients were brought to the TRAIN by box ambulances (pictured above).

(Photo courtesy of Virginia Taylor collection)

THE CHAIN OF CASUALTY EVACUATION
VIRGINIA TAYLOR'S 1956 STANFORD THESIS[33]

1. ## THE MEDICAL AID MEN (DOC)

It was the aid men, whose courage and speed in rescuing the wounded, helped make it possible for the U.S. Army Medical Corps in Korea to write an amazing new chapter in the miracles of military medicine.

He worked in a hell already too hazardous for the combat troops. During a retreat, it was the medical aid man who went after the wounded. In war, he was required to be nurse, junior doctor, chaplain, and rescue squad all at the same time. Speed was always the important factor. Minutes saved were always lives saved. They were the bravest, these unsung heroes, the medical aid men.

2. ## THE BATTALION AID STATION

The first stop for the wounded man after he received first aid was the BATTALION AID STATION. It was located anywhere from a couple of miles to a thousand yards from the front and possibly still under enemy fire, for men were occasionally hit as they lie on litters outside of the B.A. Tent. Still more lives were saved by keeping it near to the fighting; so close, in fact, that sometimes it had to move two or three times in one day to keep close to the moving battle lines.

The aid station was usually housed in a large tent. A large field chest held assorted battle dressings for any type of wound. Another chest was fitted for medicine bottles, instruments, and all the new antibiotics. A third chest carried the CO's typewriter, plus forms for recording battle casualties and supply requisitions, the minimum red tape of the Army. In the winter, it may have had a pot-bellied stove. <u>Nearby were several jeeps each fitted to carry two litters</u>. An Army doctor and several aid men processed the casualties as they came through the B.A. Tent. Blood soaked bandages were changed here and bleeding was brought under control.

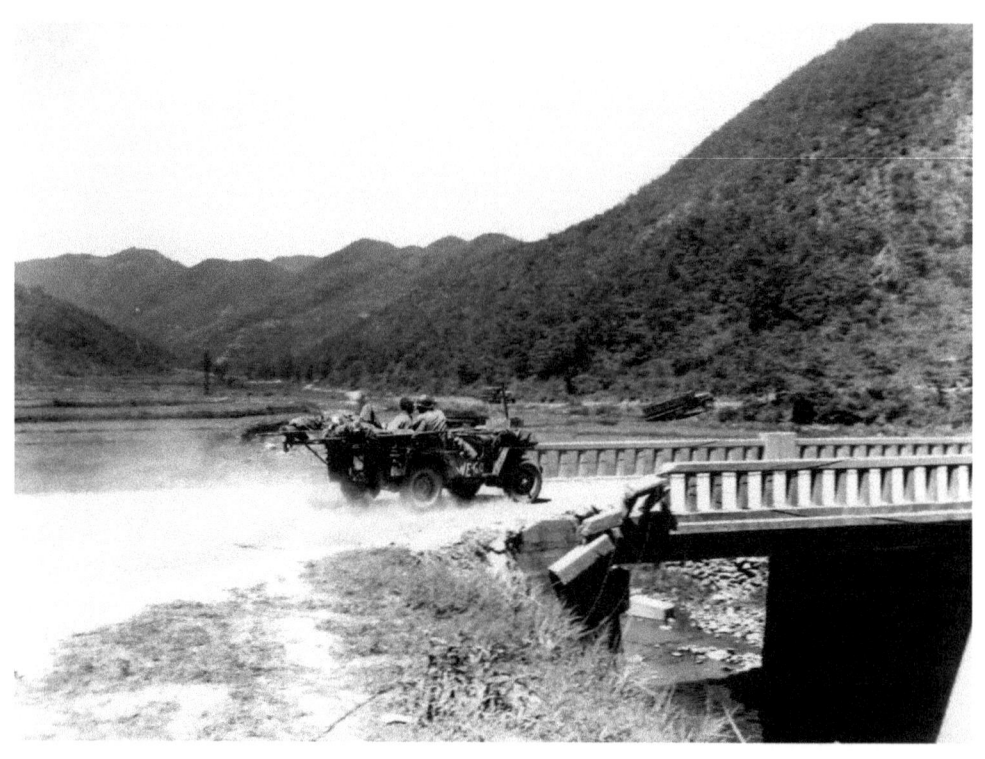

A litter-bearer team moves two wounded to an aid station[34]
(Photo courtesy of Virginia Taylor collection)

3. THE COLLECTING AND CLEARING STATIONS

The first stop after the B.A. Station was the COLLECTING STATION. This medical unit served as an important relay point where wounds could be checked and more plasma given if necessary. Sometimes this station was bypassed and the wounded man taken directly to the CLEARING STATION or MASH.

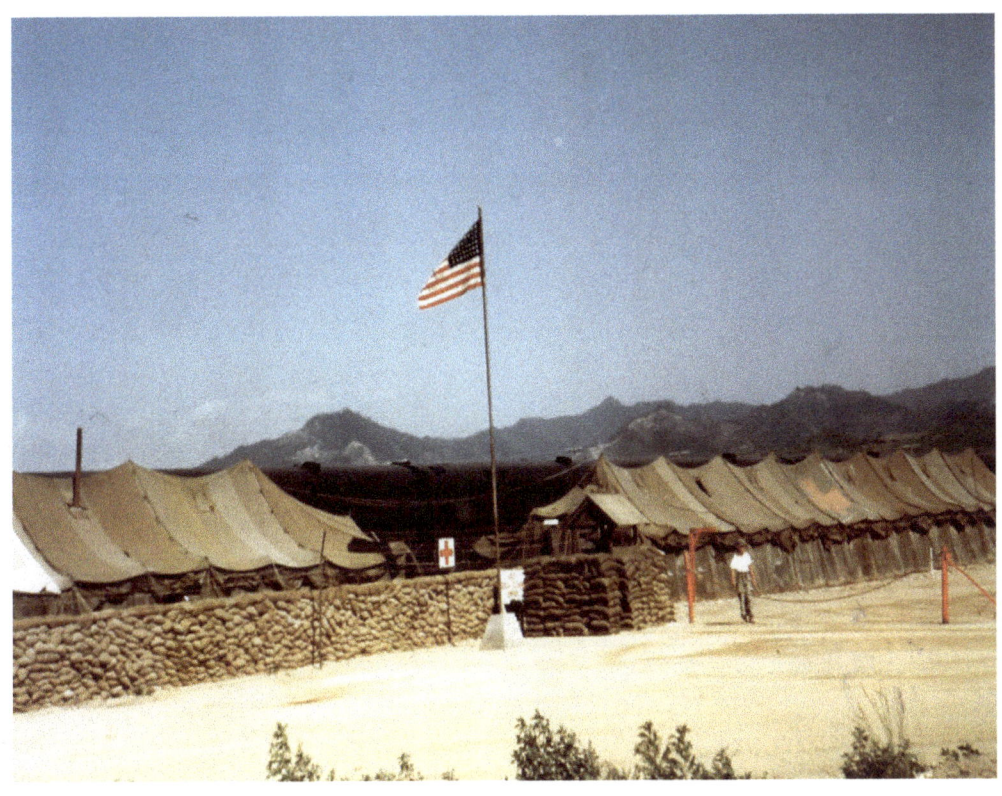

CHONKOK (618 CLEARING COMPANY STATION)

10 Miles above the 38th Parallel, North Korea
Hospital Train 105 in the background
(Photo courtesy of Virginia Taylor collection)

4. MASH (The Mobile Army Surgical Hospital)

The small MASH, a past World War II development, offered several wounded men definitive surgery shortly after they have been hurt, often within a few minutes. Located in a division area near the frontlines, the hospital received patients by helicopter and ambulance, provided them with immediate surgery and kept them until they could be safely evacuated further to the rear, usually by the HOSPITAL TRAINS.

8055th MASH (Below) The first of its kind in Korea. By October 1952, it had treated and evacuated its fifty thousandth battle casuality. The hospital personnel took pride in the amazing patient recovery rate of 99.8%.[35]

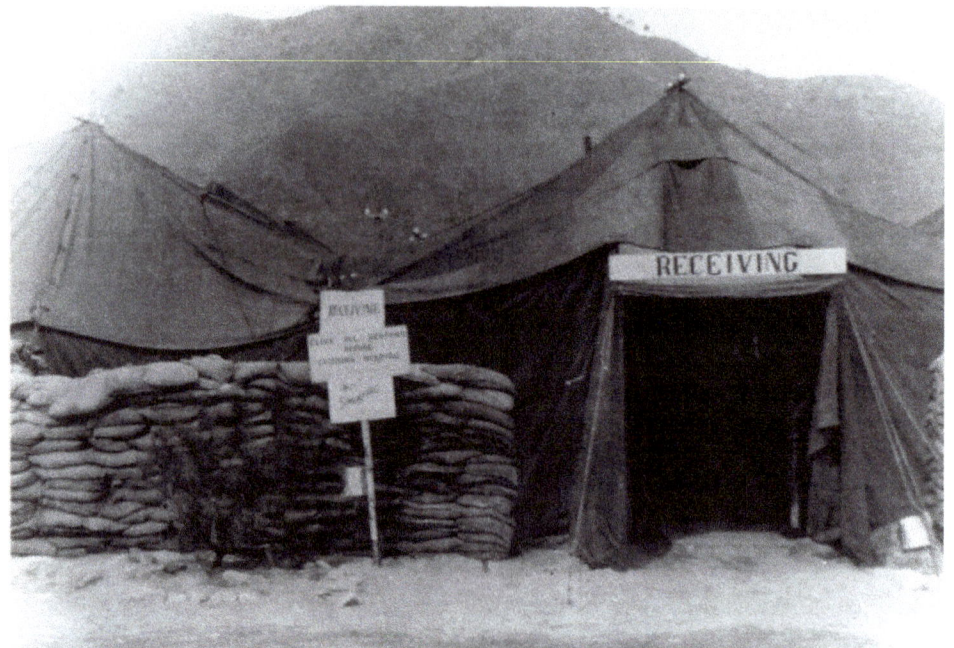

MASH 8055—FOUR miles from the CHONKOK Clearing Station.

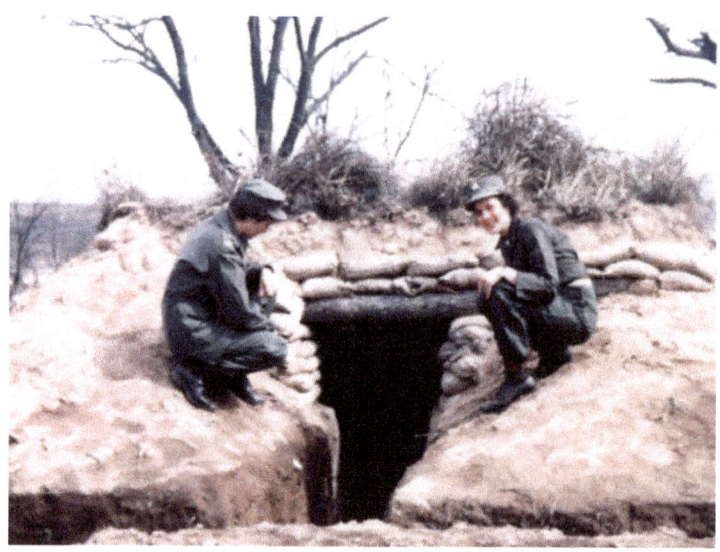

Virginia Taylor with Capt. Ruth Dixon, MASH 8055 Chief Nurse, looking at a bunker on site.

(Photos courtesy of Virginia Taylor collection)

5. THE HELICOPTERS (Choppers, Windmills, Angels)

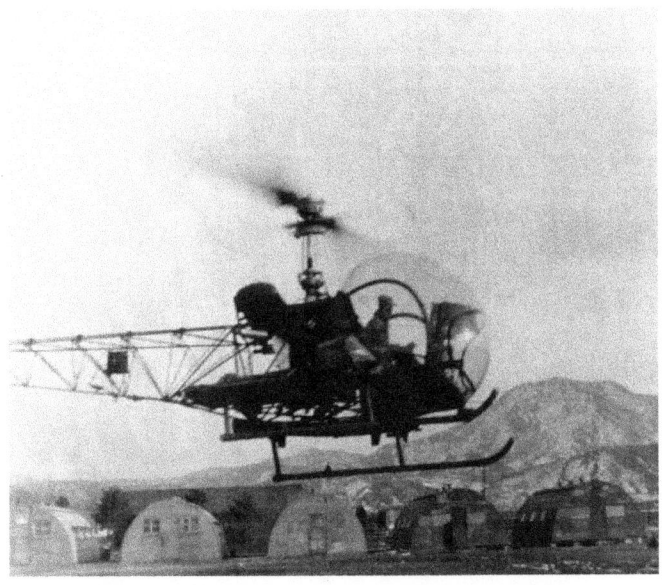

(Photo courtesy of the Virginia Taylor collection)[36]

The first helicopters were sent in by the Air Force to rescue pilots shot down behind enemy lines. With this short range and because they needed to go as deeply as possible into enemy territory, they were billeted at the MASH Units (bed, shelter and their windmills gas). In return, when there were no fallen birdman to retrieve, would do odd jobs for the MASH. Often a battalion aid station would phone in to report a case so badly wounded that he would not survive a trip in a jolting ambulance over Korea's war-chewed roads, so the chopper would retrieve him. The choppers were saving so many lives that the Army attached four of them, each carrying two litters, to each MASH unit.

6. THE HOSPITAL TRAINS (Mercy Trains)

In Korea, the hospital trains went as far forward as the Division <u>Collecting Station.</u> <u>In one location, the forward railhead was within 8,000 yards of the enemy line.</u> Many of the seriously wounded were spared the jolting ride of an ambulance with these smooth efficient hospitals on wheels.

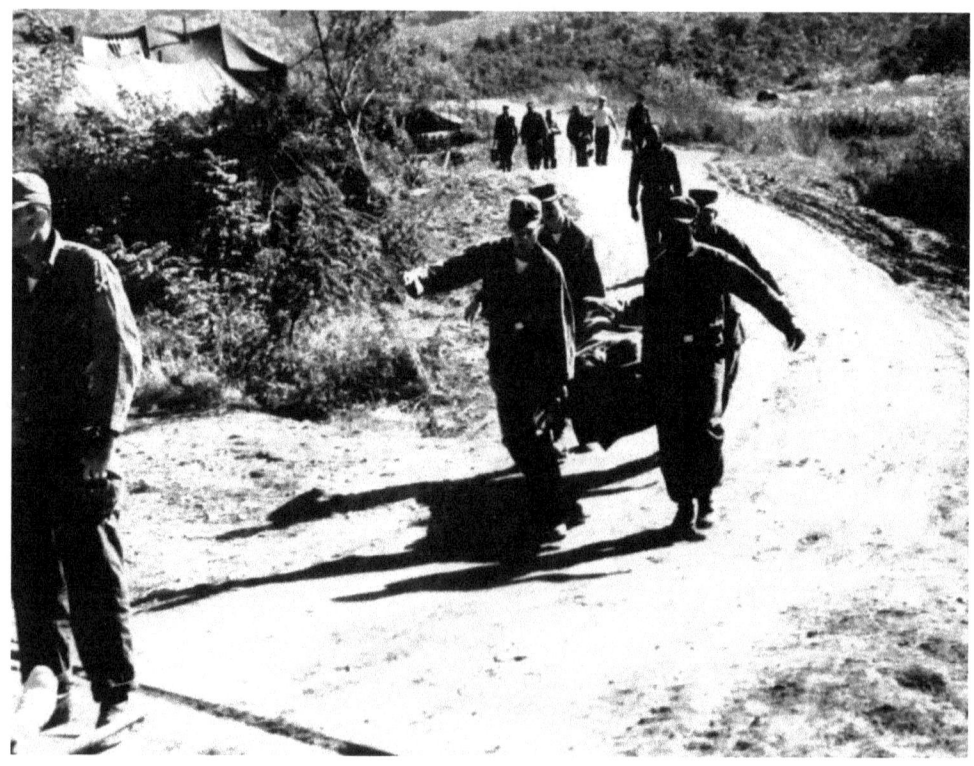

Hospital Train 105 medics carrying wounded to the train
SINTANNI COLLECTING STATION
8,000 Yards from the enemy lines

30 miles above the 38th Parallel in North Korea
(Photo courtesy of Virginia Taylor collection)

The trains moved casualties from the Collecting and Clearing Stations and MASH hospitals to the larger Evacuation Hospitals in the rear. As one train moved south, another train headed north.

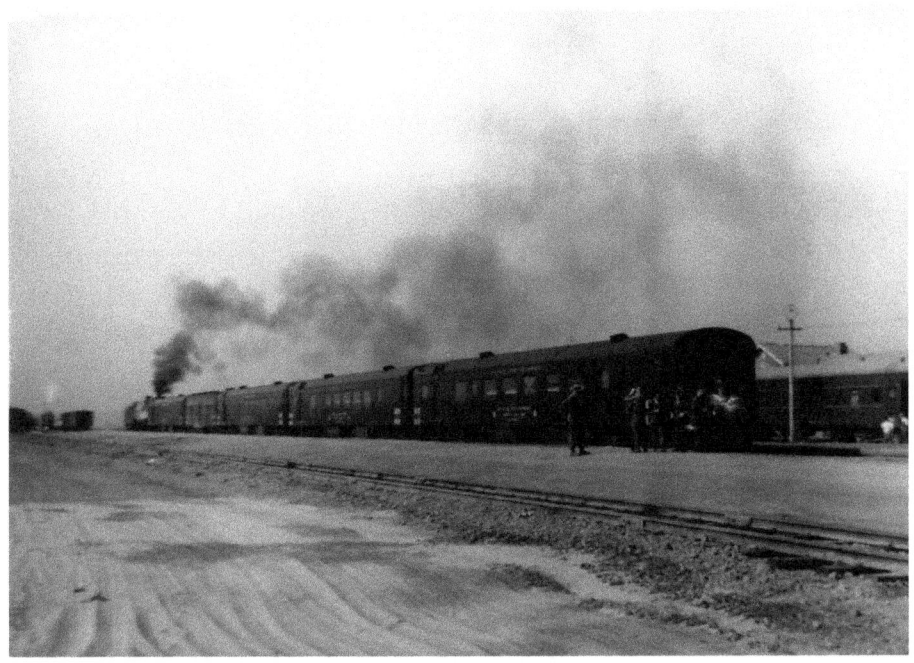

Hospital Train 105
(Photo Courtesy of Virginia Taylor collection)

There were eight individual trains (101-108) in operation throughout Korea. Each train was made up of one doctor, one nurse, and fifteen enlisted men. Each train was capable of carrying 216 bed patients, although at times during heavy fighting as many as 300 were evacuated on one train.

To operate and maintain the "Mercy Express" and to keep her on schedule with her precious "payload" were some of the BEST railroaders in the Army. Most of whom had clicked off many railroad miles on stateside commercial roads. During the long, cold Korean winter months, steam was used exclusively to provide heating facilities to the individual cars. In the summer, diesel engines furnished the power.

The hospital train or rail buses were also used to evacuate the wounded from Evacuation hospitals to the airfields where they were flown to Japan. This saved the men a jolting ambulance ride over dusty, rutted roads. (See map of Korea for routes of the hospital trains, pg 5.)

7. THE EVACUATION HOSPITAL

The Evacuation Hospitals in Korea were situated in old school houses or in one case a cotton mill. The school's auditorium served as a 100-bed general surgical ward. The halls were drab and drafty, old potbellied stoves served as the heating units and sliding doors helped keep out some of the winter air. The essentials, however, were all there. With the ingenuity and improvising of experts, the Engineers, Signal Corps, and Quartermaster, helped keep the evacuation hospital operating on much the same order as a modern stateside unit. In each evacuation hospital, there was modern operating room equipment, an up-to-date dentist office, trained X-ray men with all necessary equipment, a modern laboratory, and a central supply with autoclaves. Each had their own light and water plant.

37

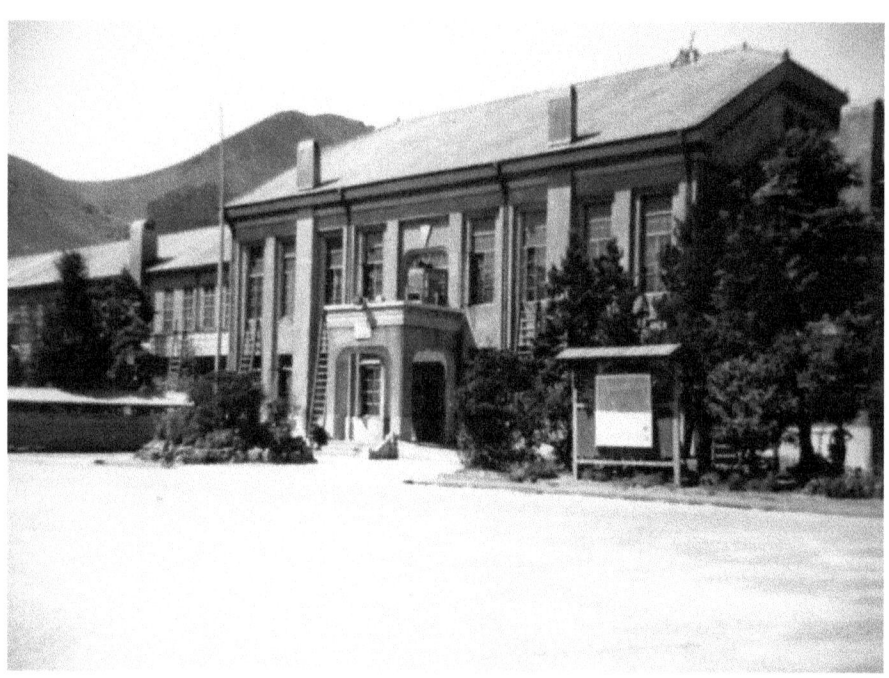

21ST EVAC HOSPITAL, PUSAN
(Old school building)
Previously, 3rd Evac Hospital

(Photo Courtesy of the Virginia Taylor collection)

The 121st Evacuation Hospital near Seoul was perhaps the largest and the best equipped of the evacuation hospitals. It had a bed capacity of over 750. The 171st Evacuation Hospital in Taejon, although staffed with American Medical Personnel, cared only for the Korean Service Corps.[38] The 11th Evacuation Hospital in Wonju was made a center for treatment of epidemic hemorrhagic fever in early 1951. Early in the war, the 21st Evacuation Hospital in Pusan handled 18,000 casualties during a three-month period— of this number, only 49 were lost.

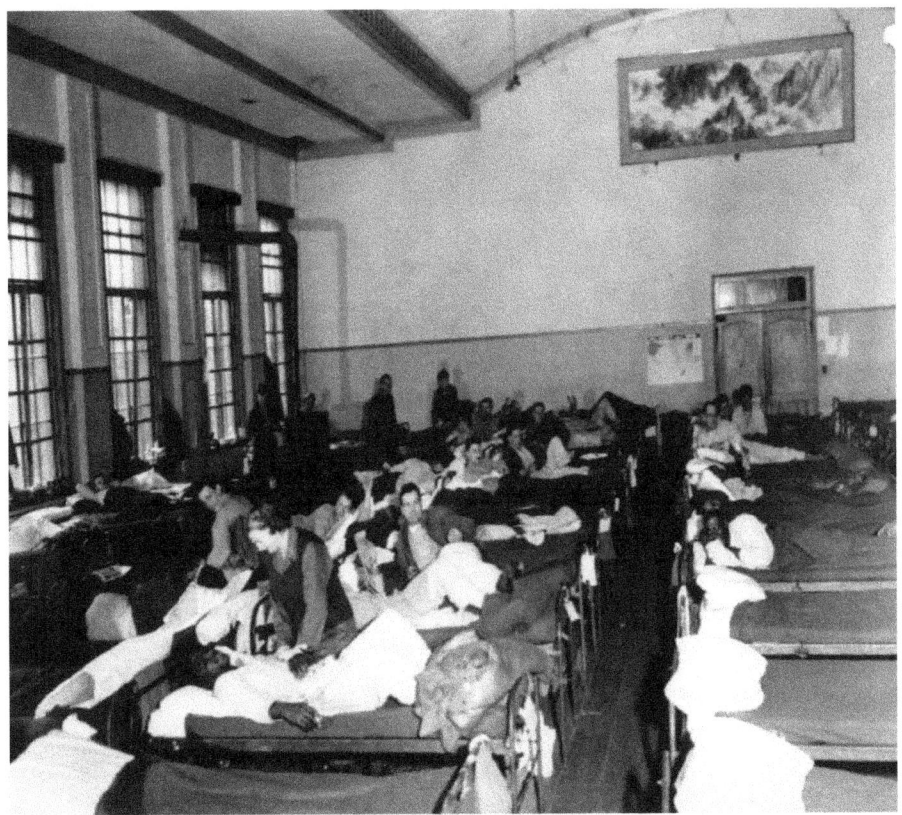

21ST EVAC HOSPITAL, PUSAN
(Old school building)
(Photo courtesy of the Virginia Taylor collection)[39]

(All of the hospital train nurses lived at the 21st EVAC Hospital when not on the trains)

8. HOSPITAL SHIPS

To the physician and surgeon of our armed forces, Navy and Army working side by side, an injured man was a patient, be he infantryman, artilleryman, airman, or marine, or even an enemy soldier. The extent of the man's injury, not rank or service, determined the treatment he received.

Three Navy hospital ships: the *Consolation, Haven,* and *Repose* operated alternately in and about the waters of the Korean coast. When one was in Korea, another was in Japan, and the other enroute home to the United States. These floating 700-bed hospitals were as spacious and well-equipped as anything one could find back in the United States and better than most. All three of the ships were fitted with helicopter decks and carried their own "whirlybirds."

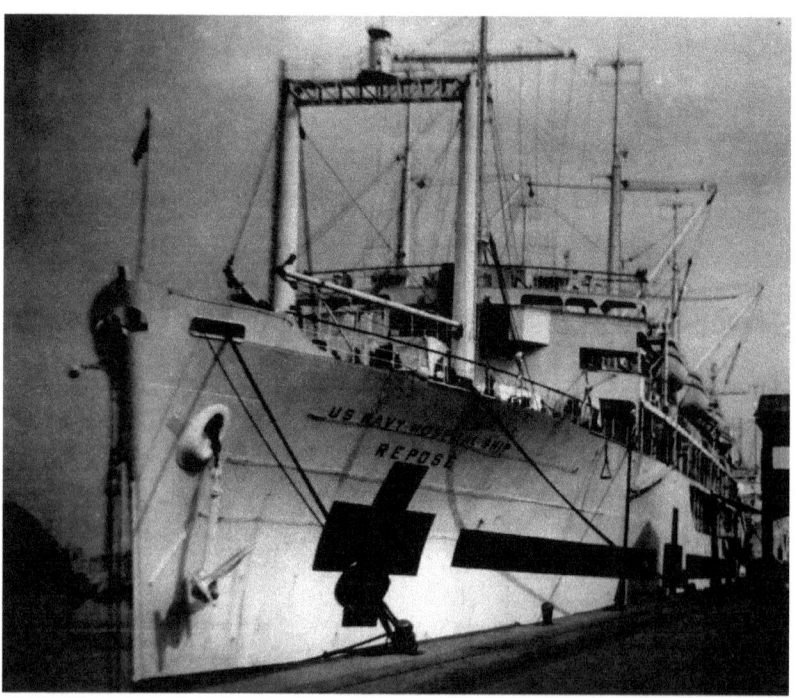

REPOSE HOSPITAL SHIP
Pusan Harbor
(Photo courtesy of Virginia Taylor collection)

The Danish hospital ship, *Jutlandia,* also was assigned to Korean waters. It had a bed capacity of 300 and a medical and administrative staff of 100. During its 16-months of intensive duty off Korea, its medical staff assisted thousands of patients—young and old, civilian and military, from the Republic of Korea and the various forces fighting under the United Nation's command.

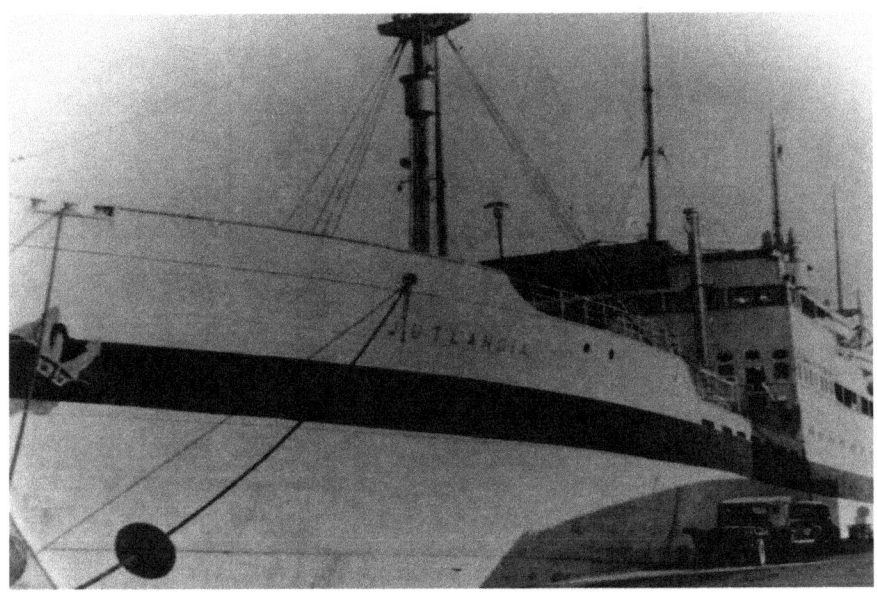

JUTLANDIA HOSPITAL SHIP
(Photo courtesy of Virginia Taylor collection)

9. <u>MILITARY AIR TRANSPORT SERVICE (MATS)</u>

From the evacuation hospital, the seriously sick or wounded soldier was further evacuated by the Military Air Transport Service to large, modern hospitals in Japan, approximately one hour and a-half away. As each litter case was brought aboard the MATS transport, the flight nurse checked their wounds and records. Contagious diseases went up front. Men with heavy hip casts and leg wounds were arranged so their casts rested on the aisle side of the plane. Men with frozen hands and feet were placed where their arms and legs could be raised and lowered at intervals. Men with throat and face injuries had to be checked so they could be fed through a tube. There were no doctors on these flights. The nurse and two or three medical technicians handled the men alone.

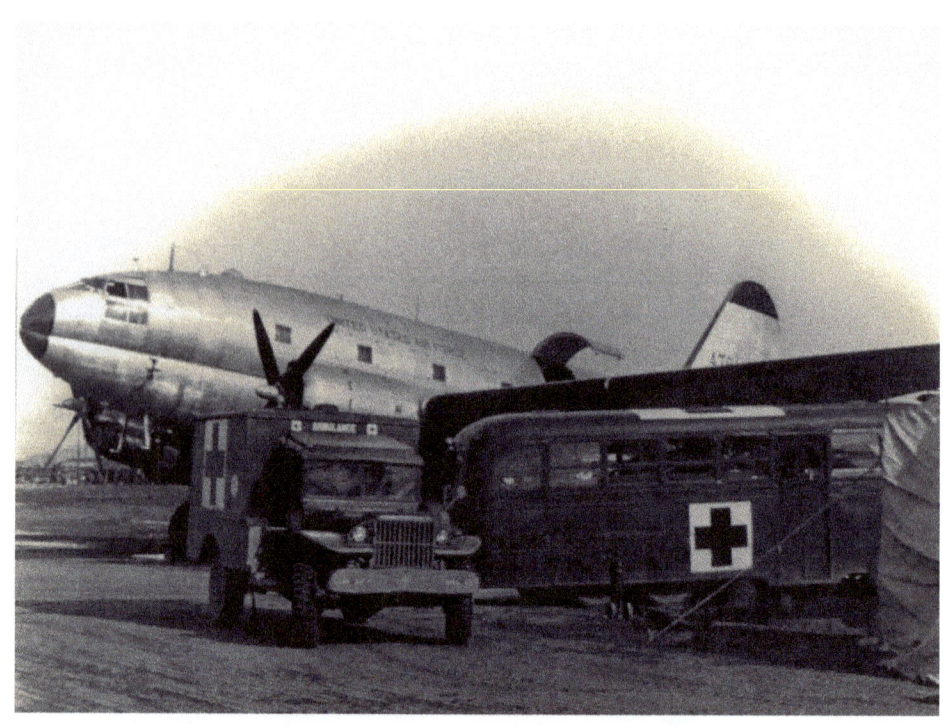
Military Air Transport Service (MATS)
(Photo courtesy of the Virginia Taylor collection)

DON VERSTRAETE'S RECOLLECTION
(Medic/Car Commander - Train 106 from 1952-1953)

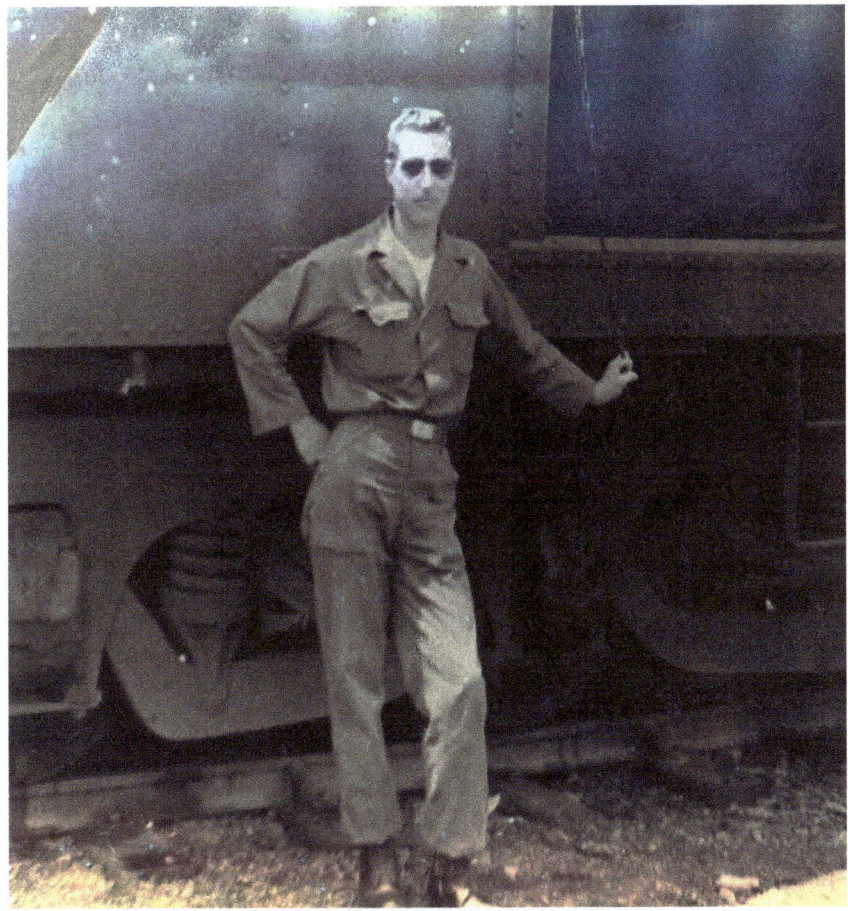

Don Verstraete, Medic and Car Commander, Train 106
8138th AU Hospital Trains. Korea

(Photo courtesy of Don Verstraete collection)

All eight trains were stationed at Pusan Harbor. Each train had a doctor and nurse who lived offsite, boarded the day of departure, and occupied one of the car's private compartments.

The enlisted men lived on their assigned train full time. These included the medics (car commanders), crew chief, mess sergeant, two cooks, and at least one to two corpsmen per car.

- <u>The Crew Chief</u> was assigned to a standard hospital train and in charge of all of the enlisted men on the train. Prior to departure, he inspected all of the cars. He also maintained the logbooks and assisted the nurse during routine checks of all the patients aboard.

- <u>A Car Commander</u> (Medic) assigned to the 421st Medical Unit was loaned for one year to a standard hospital train. He was in charge of his car, the corpsmen, and all the patients under his care.

- <u>The Mess Sergeant</u> was the chief cook and kitchen supervisor. He also ensured that all provisions were in place before the train departed. He and the cooks assigned to a standard hospital train lived aboard full time.

- Two train engineers and technicians also lived aboard. A Korean Interpreter and MPs accompanied each trip.

- The standard train consisted of seven cars: Six Pullman-type ward cars and one kitchen/dining car. (<u>A total of 216 beds per train</u>.)

- Each car accommodated <u>thirty-six patients</u>. The loading of the three-tier berths in the main cabin would start at the top, middle, and then bottom. Six berths at the back section were used by the live-in crew when the train was not transporting wounded.

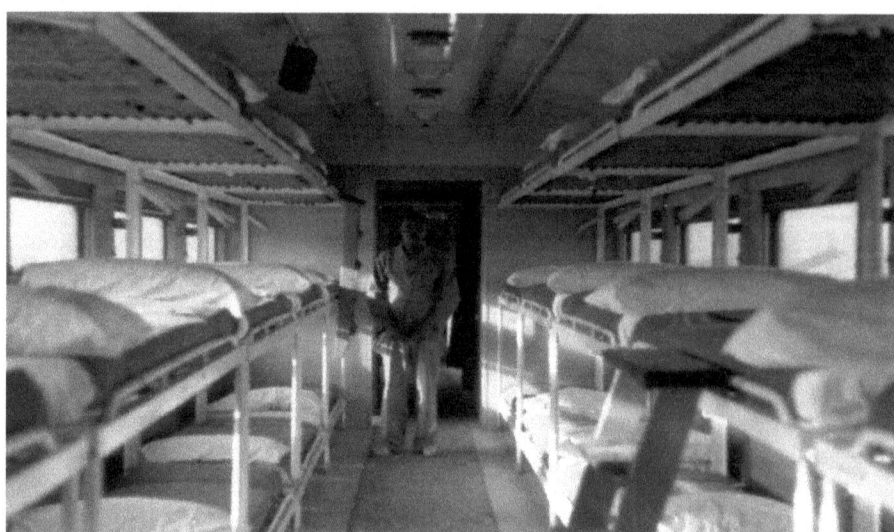

(Photo courtesy Virginia Taylor) Train 105

- On one end of the car were two private compartments with pull-down bunks. When the bunks were up, there was a desk and chair for the occupant to use. (Don occupied one of the compartments on his car and the cook lived in the other.)

- Near the private compartments were a lavatory, sink, and shower. Behind the shower were storage bins for the crew. At the end of each car was a vestibule with side double-doors for loading and unloading litters.

- One kitchen/dining/pharmacy car was located in the middle of the train with three hospital ward-cars on each side.

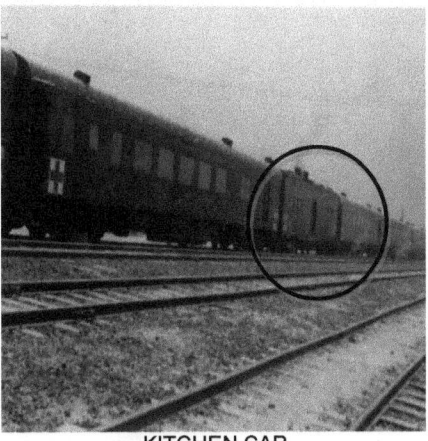

KITCHEN CAR
(Photo courtesy of Virginia Taylor collection)
Train 105

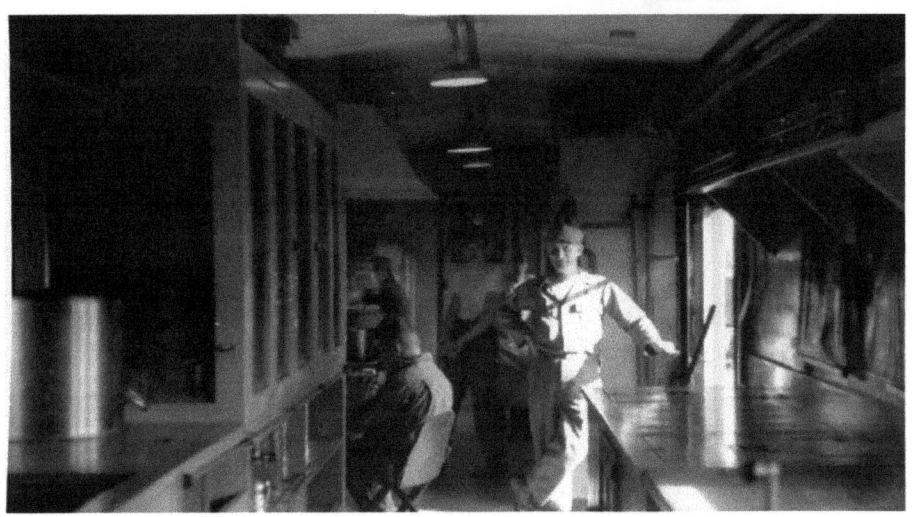

HOSPITAL TRAIN KITCHEN-DINING-PHARMACY CAR Train 105
(Photo courtesy of Virginia Taylor collection)

- The kitchen cars were converted from baggage cars and self-contained with hot and cold water, electrical, and a coal-fired stove and oven.

- Don's train 106 had two cooks (one of the cooks was the Mess Sergeant). Hot food was served once during the trip. Usually meat and potatoes and sometimes dessert. Coffee was available throughout the trip. All meals were served on metal trays (no plates) and tin cups. Don's car was the farthest back. He had to travel through two cars to get to the kitchen.

- The car commander and two corpsmen would pick up the trays from the kitchen car and distribute the meals, then return the empty trays to the kitchen. The kitchen car also had a dining area for sitting.

- Most of the wounded on Train 106 were ambulatory South Korean soldiers.

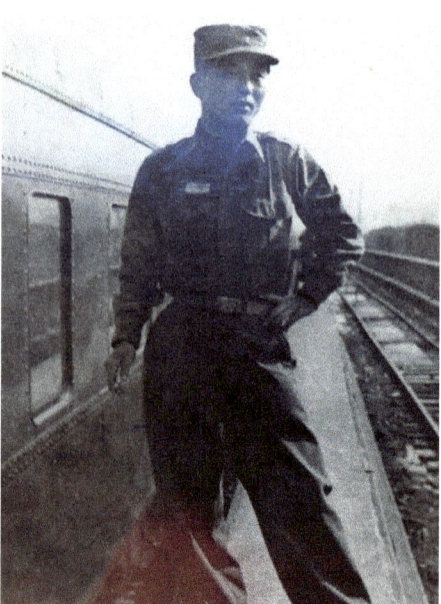

Mr. Shim, TRAIN 106 Interpreter
(Photo courtesy of Don Verstraete collection)

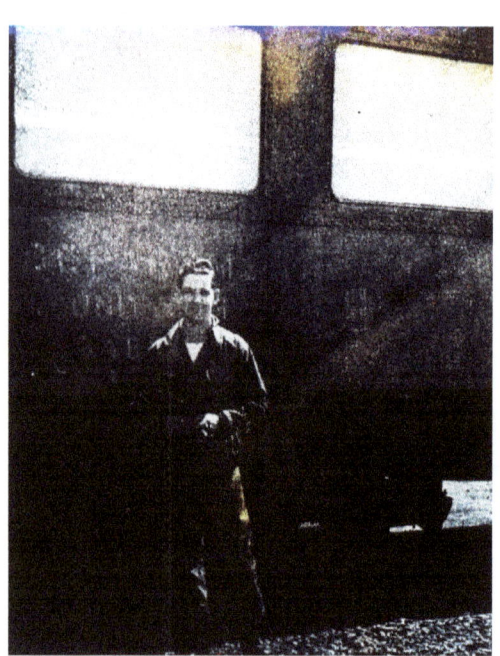

Medic/Car Commander Jack Roth
TRAIN 106
(Photo courtesy Don Verstraete collection)

TRAIN MAP WITH "KEY" MARKINGS
(Map by Ruth Taylor for Virginia Taylor's 1956 Stanford Thesis)

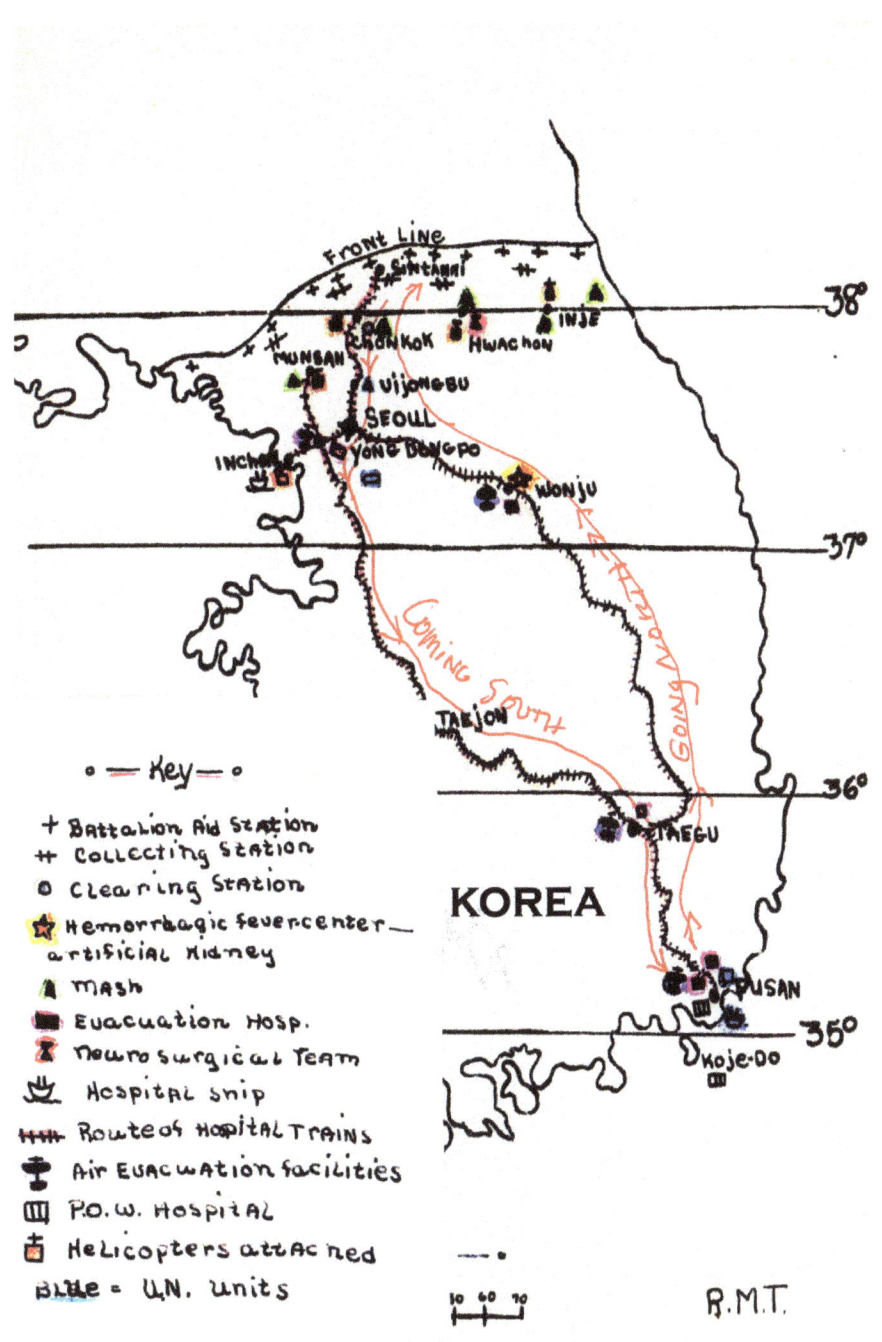

(Virginia Taylor collection) (Courtesy of

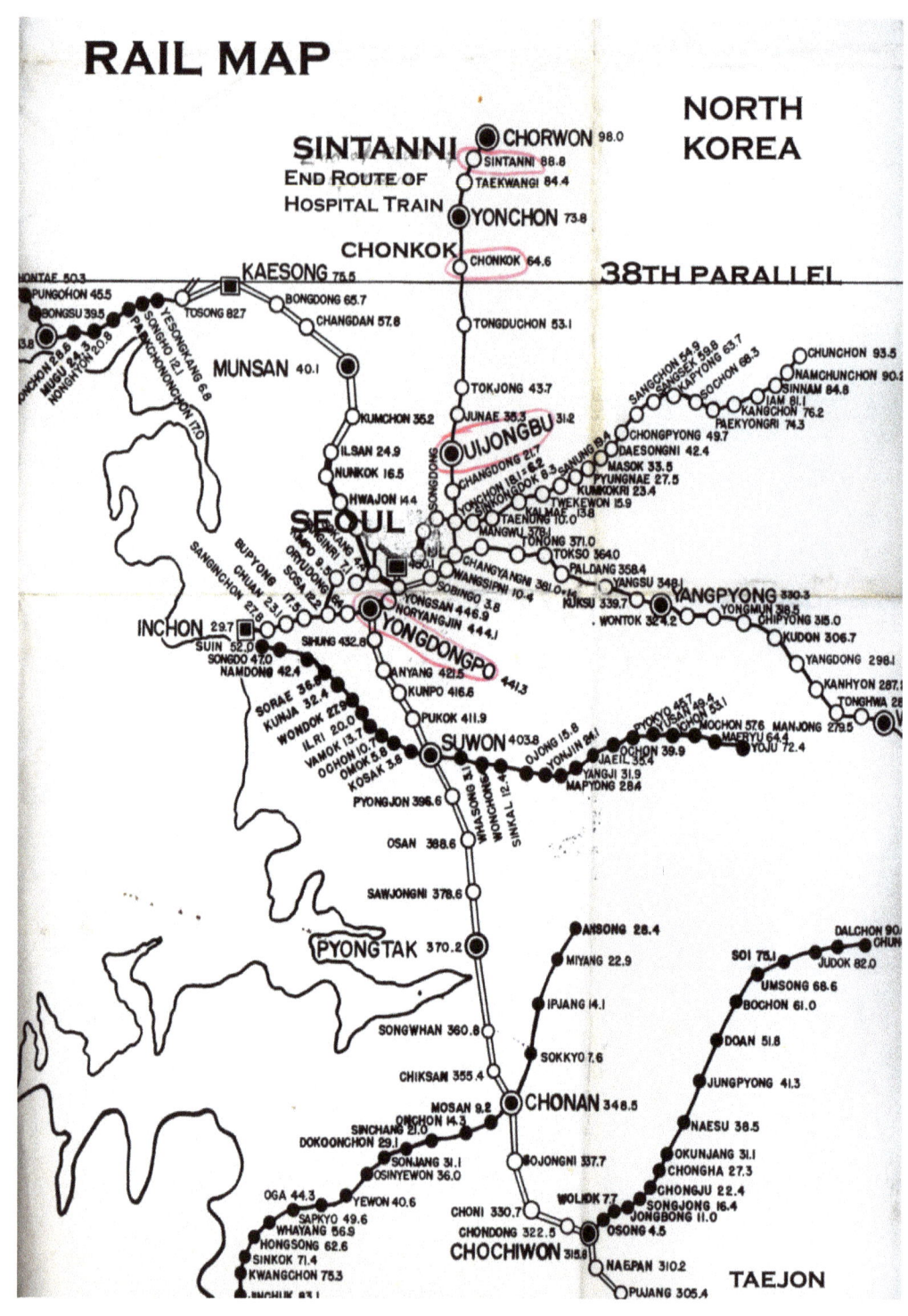

(Courtesy of Virginia Taylor collection)

ORIGINAL "KEY" SHEET USED BY VIRGINIA TAYLOR ON HOSPITAL TRAIN 105
(Courtesy of Virginia Taylor collection)

Key

- ✚ Battalion Aid Station
- ⊕ Collecting Station
- ⊖ Clearing Station
- ☆ Hemorrhagic Fever Center - Artificial Kidney
- △ MASH
- ▢ Evacuation Hosp.
- ◆ Neurosurgical Team
- ◯ Respirators
- ⚓ Hospital Ships
- ⎯⎯⎯ Route of Hospital Trains
- ✈ Air Evacuation Facilities
- ▥ P.O.W. Hospital
- ⌂ Helicopter Attached

Pusan - 21st Evac. ~~500 beds~~ - Respirator
 22nd Evac. ~~500~~ Respirator
 Swedish Evac. ~~500~~
 Jutlandia Danish Hosp. Ship 400
 3rd & 14th Field POW Hosp.

Kojedo - 64th Field POW Hosp.

Taegu - 25th Evac - Respirator

Taejon - 171st Evac - Respirator

WonJu - 117th Evac - Hemorrhagic Fever Center Respirator Artificial Kidney

Inchon - Consolation - Repose or Haven Alternating USNHS Hospital Ships - 700 beds - Caring for Wounded of 1st Marines

Youngdongpo - 121st Evac - 1000 beds - Respirator

Munsan - MASH 1st Marine
~~Uijongbu - Norwegian MASH~~
Chonkok - 618 Clearing
 8055 MASH

Hwachon - 8063 MASH - Neurological unit Attached

Inje - 8076 MASH

(This for my use)

In addition to battlefield injuries, Hemorrhagic Fever and other diseases (malaria, typhus, etc.) were a concern too. Certain EVAC hospitals specialized in the treatments as referenced on Virginia's "KEY" Sheet.

Oppressive summer heat multiplied insects, and impure water brought obvious sources of disease, but fleas from rodents were a universal plague. Patients evacuated from the frontline were often infested, as were the doctors, nurses, and attendants working over them. DDT dusting and spraying of clothing, beds, billets and hospital wards and trains began. [40] Hemorrhagic Fever was transmitted by mites from a common field rodent.[41] Lice in the trenches could transmit typhus, trench fever, and epidemic relapsing fever.

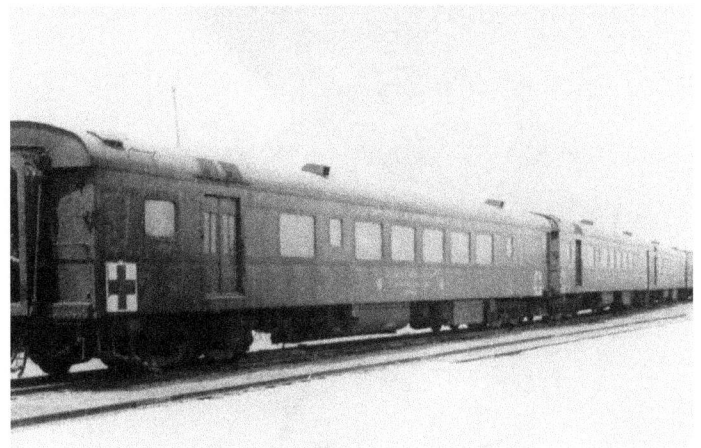
TRAIN 106
(Photo courtesy Don Verstraete collection)

DON VERSTRAETE
(Medic/Car Commander - Train 106 (1952-1953)

HOSPITAL TRAIN ROUTINE

Each of the eight trains (101-108) followed a similar schedule. Usually as one train headed north, another was pulling into the station with wounded. There was a daily cycle of incoming and outgoing hospital trains.

- DAY ONE: Don's train 106 departed Pusan at approximately 10:00 a.m. to Yongdongpo. The cutoff NORTH was at Taegu. (See map.) With no stops, this trip took approximately twelve hours.

  - One hour after departure, the doctor, nurse, and crew chief would inspect the car. After that, the medics and corpsmen were on their own.
  - From noon until bed (approx. 10:30 p.m.), Don and another medic friend plus two others would put up a card table and play double-pack pinochle. (The cards were provided by the Red Cross.)
  - Don and corpsmen usually ate in their own car, in the vestibule section.

- DAY TWO: In Yongdongpo (near Seoul), the crew rested or got off to sightsee. Both engines were unhooked and taken to the RR yard for inspection and maintenance.

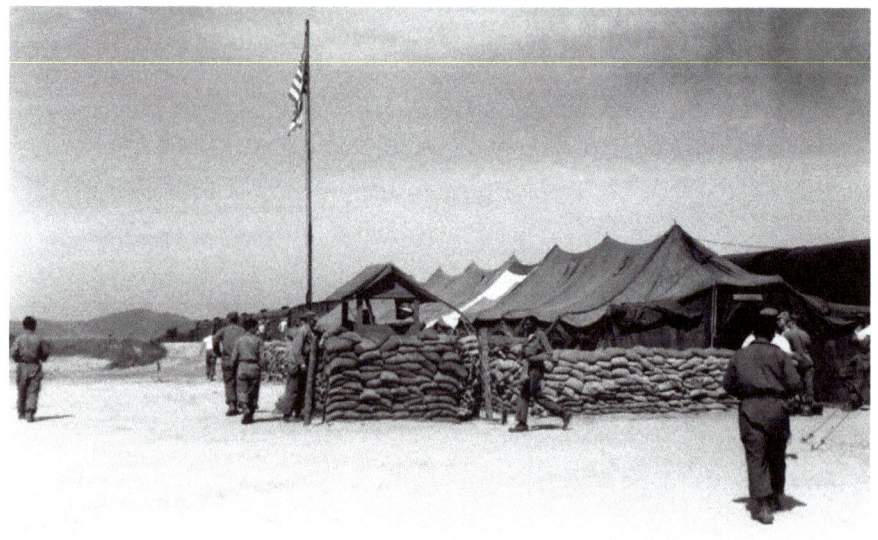

CHONKOK CLEARING STATION
Hospital Train on the right
(Photo courtesy of Virginia Taylor collection)

- DAY THREE: Mid-morning the cars were hooked up to an engine, but not the original engines. Train 106 headed north over the 38th parallel to the 618th Clearing Company CHONKOK Station, North Korea, and loaded South Korean wounded onto the train. They were brought back to the Yongdongpo Station, then transported by ambulance to the 121st EVAC Hospital.

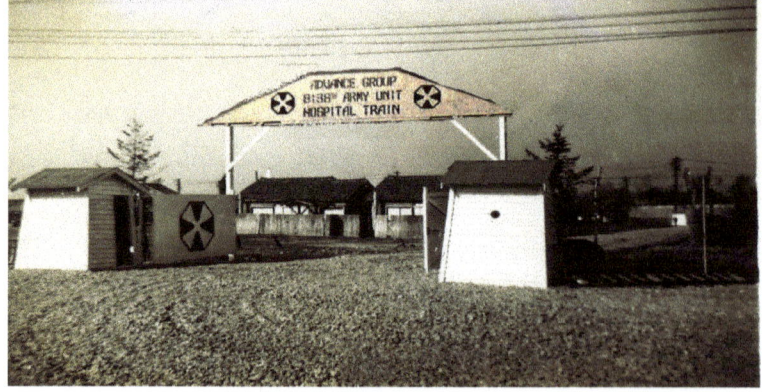

Yongdongpo Station
(Photo courtesy of Virginia Taylor collection)

- DAY FOUR: Mid-morning, Train 106 headed north again to the Chonkok Clearing Station for more South Korean patients and brought them back to Yongdongpo where they were transported by ambulance to the 121st EVAC Hospital. While there, recovering wounded, some from the previous day, were loaded into the ambulances and brought back to the train for the trip south. Room at the 121st EVAC Hospital had to be available for more incoming on the next train.

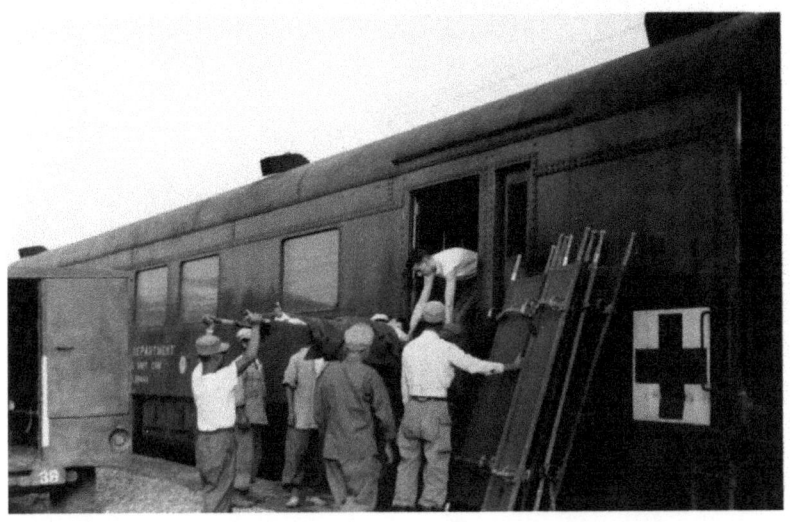

YONGDONGPO—Patients from the 121st Evac Hospital, some from the previous day, are loaded onto TRAIN 105 for the trip south.
(Photos courtesy Virginia Taylor collection)

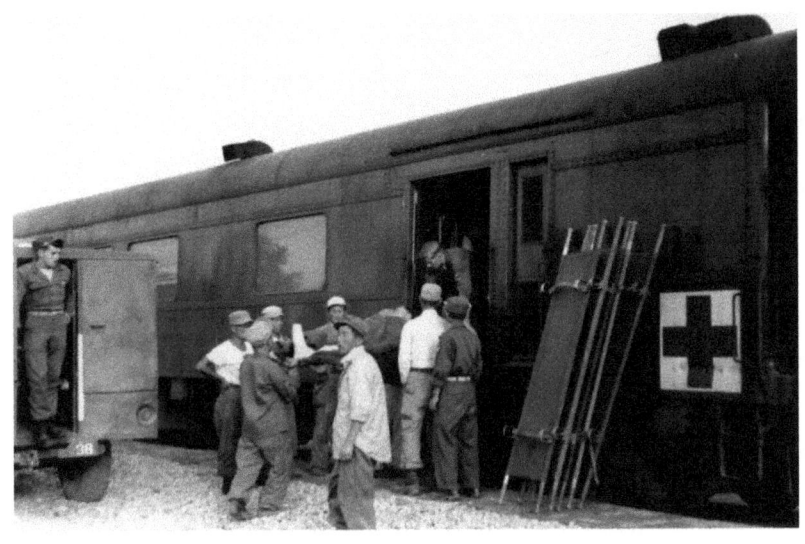

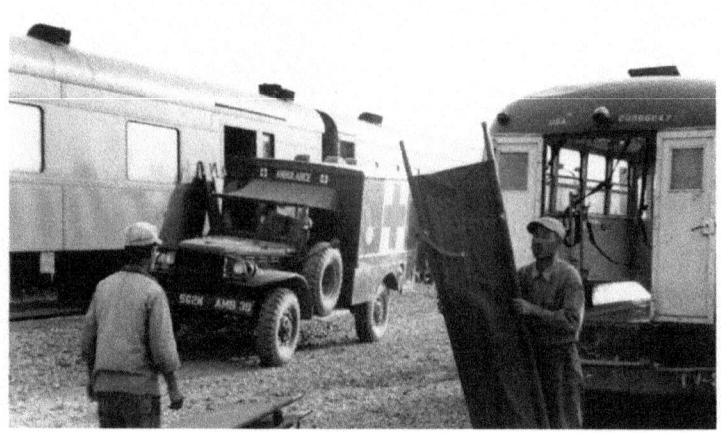
YONGDONGPO. Patients now loaded and ready for the trip south.
(Photo courtesy of Virginia Taylor collection)

- The train left Yongdongpo approx. 4:00 p.m.
- One hot meal was served on this trip.
- The train would stop at Taejon and Taegu to drop off/pick up patients at the field hospitals.[42] They would continue onto Pusan with the remaining to be transported to hospitals, hospital ships, or airfields.
- The train medics/corpsmen got little sleep on these return trips.

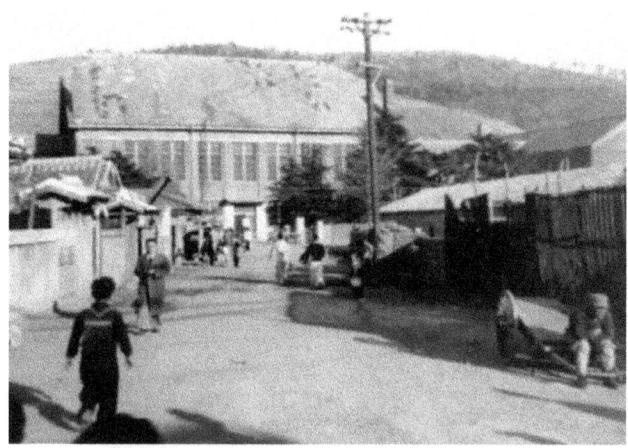
TAEGU—4th Field Hospital (old school)
(Photo courtesy Virginia Taylor collection)

- **DAY FIVE:** Train 106 would pull into Pusan early morning, between 2-4 a.m. Mid-morning, the train was taken to the wash rack to be cleaned by young Korean boys. Most of the crew stayed aboard and rested. The doctor and nurse went back to their quarters at the 21st EVAC Hospital.

  - All the linens, pillows, and blankets pulled and washed.
  - Mattresses brushed and cleaned.
  - Floors mopped.
  - The entire process for the whole train took one day (5-6 hours).
  - At least one crew member was aboard each car when the cleaning was done to watch and inspect "all" work.
  - When the cars were sprayed with DDT, the crew left for at least four hours to eat at the Army barracks.
  - The cars were then transported back to the Pusan dock, and the two engines taken to the railroad yard for maintenance.

- **DAY SIX:** The cars were reloaded with supplies. The mess sergeant supervised the loading of all non-perishable food provisions. The nurse supervised medical supplies and medicine. The car commander (medic) supervised extra needed items (blankets, etc.) on their cars. Prior to departure, a final inspection was performed by the nurse, crew chief, car commanders, and mess sergeant. Last minute food and supplies was also loaded.

The train ALWAYS had to be ready to leave on a moment's notice.

EXCERPT FROM VIRGINIA TAYLOR'S JULY 1952 LETTER TO HER PARENTS:

The days are pretty much routine as are the weeks and months. Head north for Chonkok, load up with patients, come south with patients, stay in Pusan 3 or 4 days and head north again for another load of wounded battle-weary men.

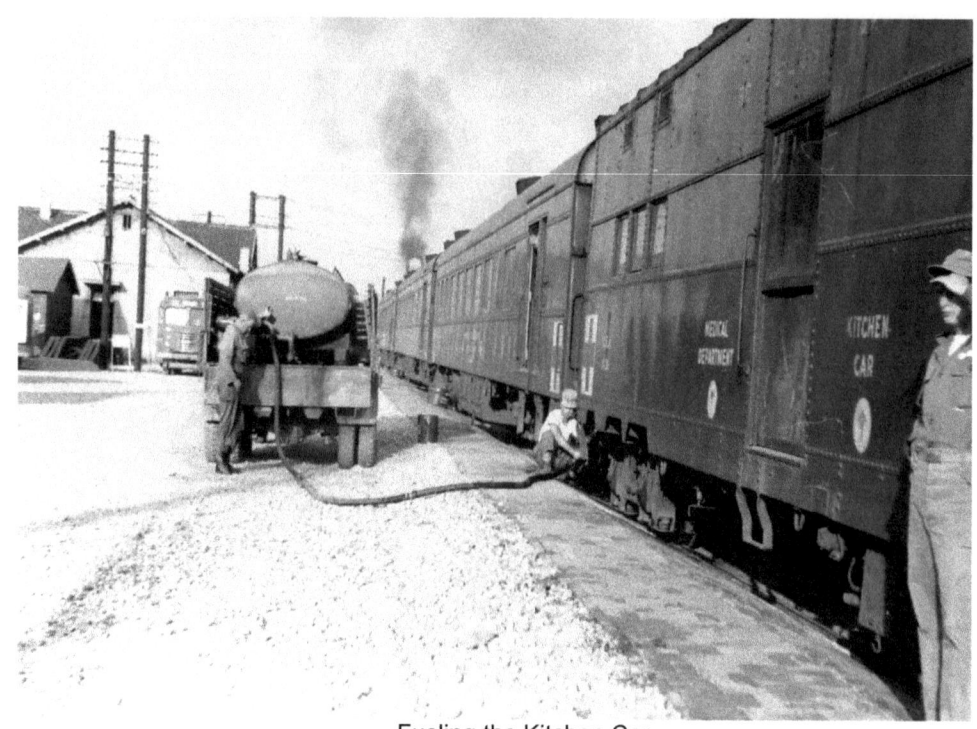

Fueling the Kitchen Car
(Hospital Train 105)

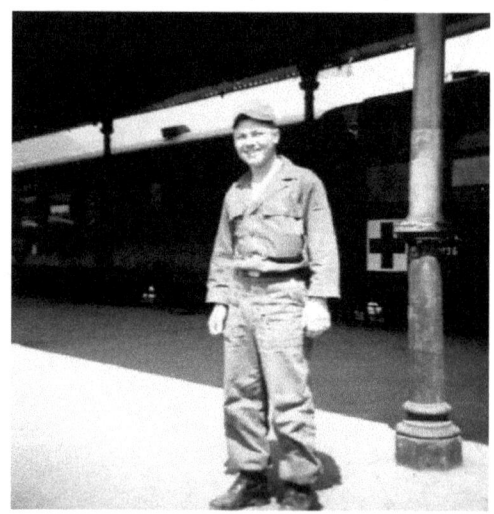

Mess Sgt Englebyecht (Train 105)
Insured that all non-perishable food provisions
were preloaded

PUSAN STATION
(Photos courtesy of Virginia Taylor collection)

NURSES OF THE 8138TH ARMY UNIT HOSPITAL TRAINS
(1951-1953)

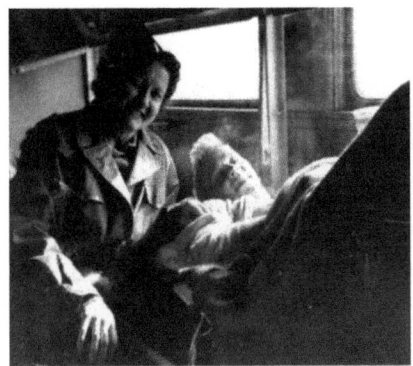

Lt. Wade (TRAIN 101)

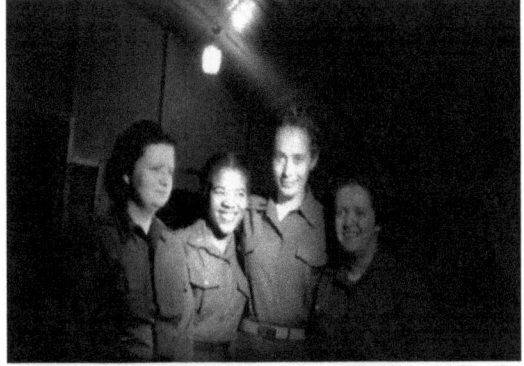

Capt. Josephine LoCicero (TRAIN 102) the "BOSS" with Lt. Virginia Taylor and two (nurse) hospital train trainees

8138 AU Train Nurses
Train 101: Lt. Wade
Train 102: Capt. LoCicero
Train 103: Lt. Potocik
Train 104: Lt. Lanternier
Train 105: Lt Taylor
Train 106: Unsure
Train 107: Unsure
Train 108: Capt. Toole

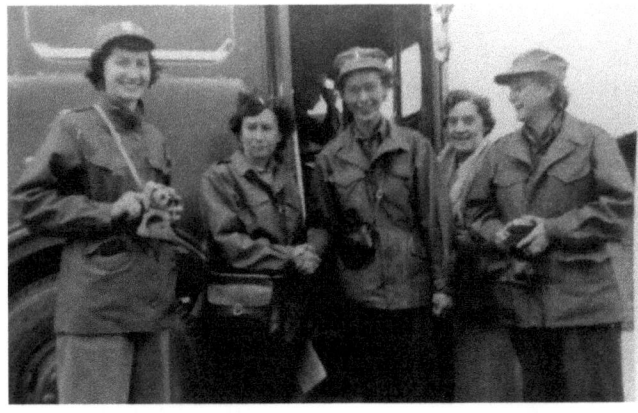

LtoR: Capt. Lena Toole   Train 108
      Lt. Betty Potocik   Train 103
      Lt. Virginia Taylor   Train 105
      Lt. Charlotte Lanternier   Train 104

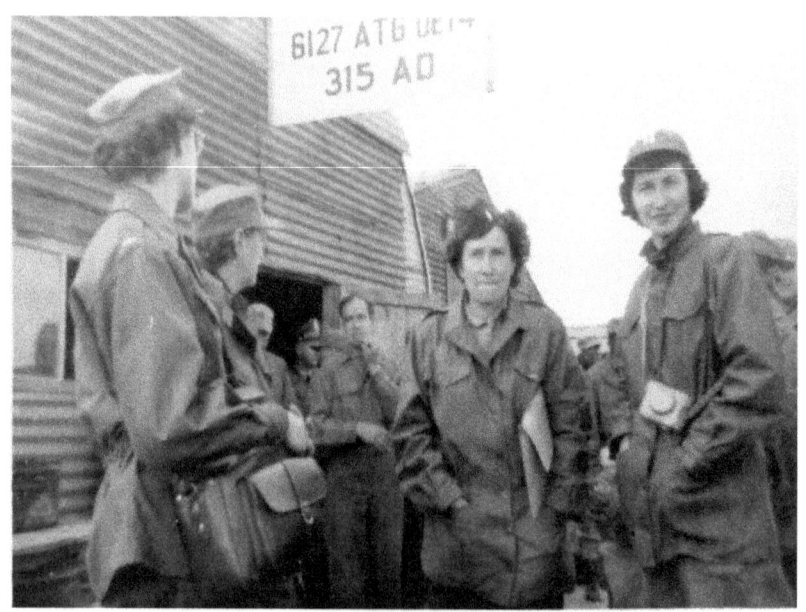

Lt. Taylor, Lt. Lanternier, Lt. Potocik, Capt. Toole

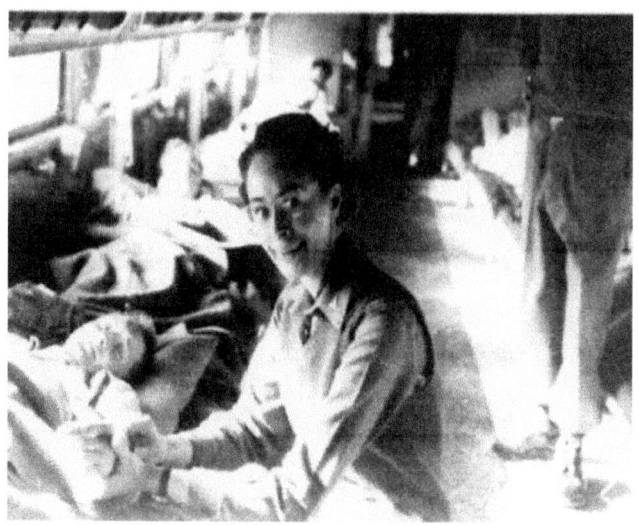

1st Lt. Virginia Taylor with patient

(Photos courtesy Virginia Taylor collection)

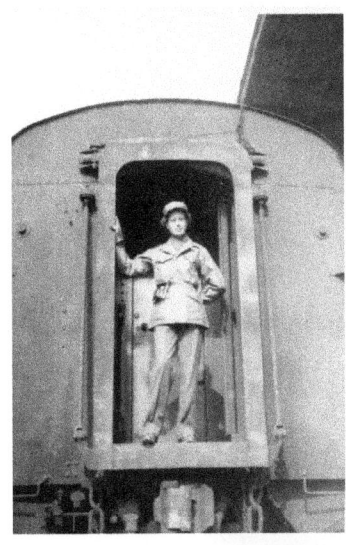

Train 105 Nurse
Lt. Virginia Taylor

(Photos courtesy of
Virginia Taylor
collection)

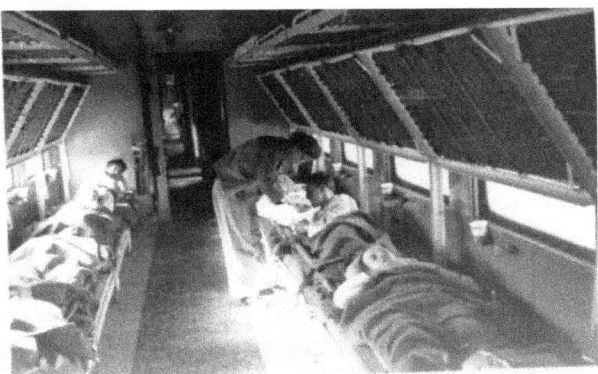

Train 108 Nurse Capt. Toole helping patient

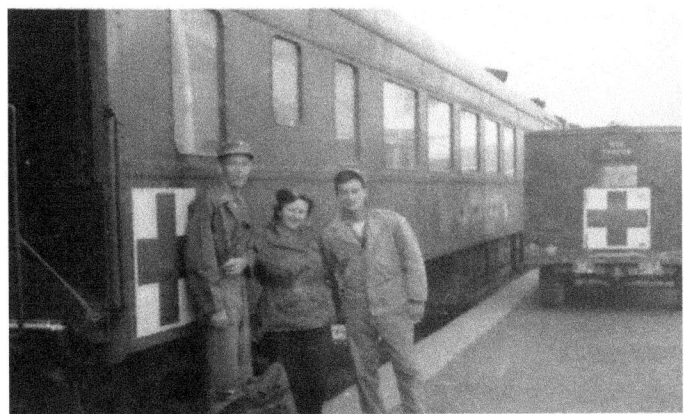

Train 101 Doctor, Nurse Lt. Wade, and Medic

From the comparative ease of modern Army hospitals, Army nurses were rushed to Korea scarcely ten days after our troops were in action. They made jet-like transition from the gentle lady in white to the sturdy woman in combat clothes who could pitch a tent as well as any male soldier.[43] They had to be combat ready.

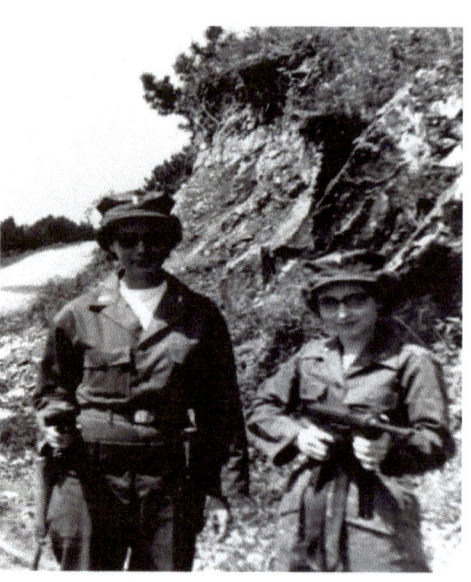

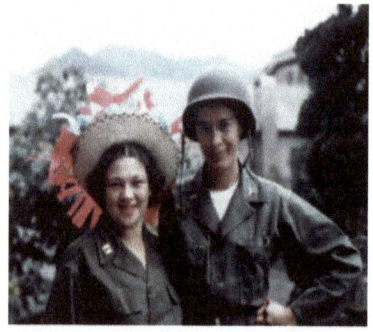

Lts. Corrine Bryant and Virginia Taylor

Lts. Virginia Taylor and Evelyn Kropp with rifle and handgun. (Virginia received her firearm training at Ft. Sam Houston, San Antonio, Texas.)

(Photos courtesy of Virginia Taylor collection)

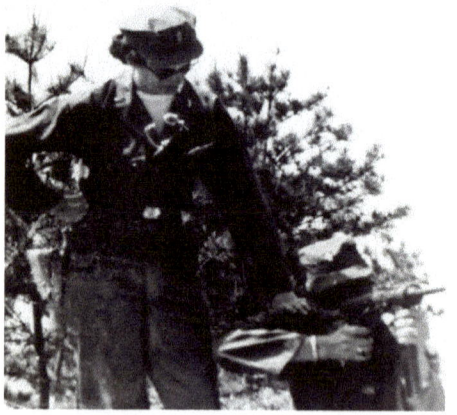

Lts. Virginia Taylor and Evelyn Kropp

THE DOCTORS

Doctors were not assigned to a particular train. Many times when a doctor was not available, Virginia Taylor served as the Train Commander for Train 105.

Captain Bauer (DOC)

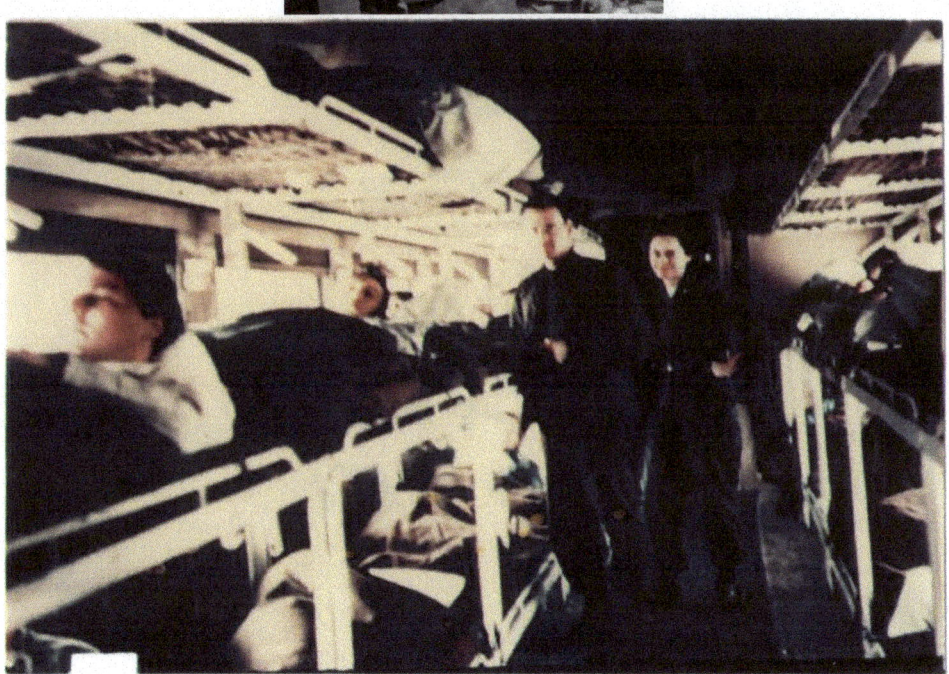

TRAIN 105 Captain (Doctor) Hukill and Nurse Virginia Taylor
(Christmas 1951)

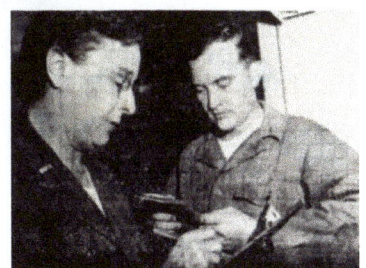

TRAIN 104 Nurse Charlotte Lanternier
and Lt (Doctor) James Meyer

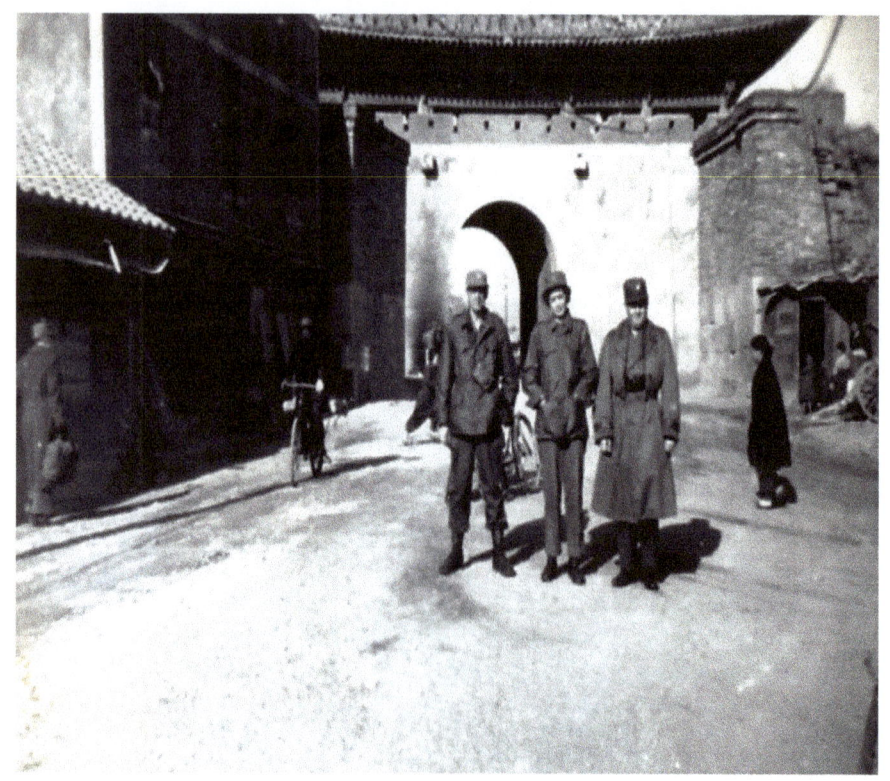

SEOUL GATE: Virginia with DOCTORS: Captain Findley and Lt. Mounee
(Photo courtesy of Virginia Taylor collection)

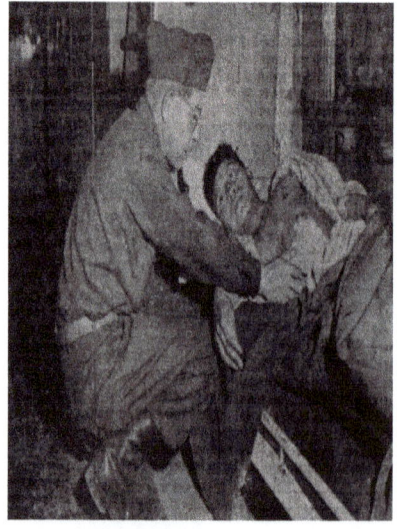

8138 AU HOSPITAL TRAIN COMMANDER
Captain (Doctor) Gerhard Newerla

HOSPITAL TRAIN 105 CREW

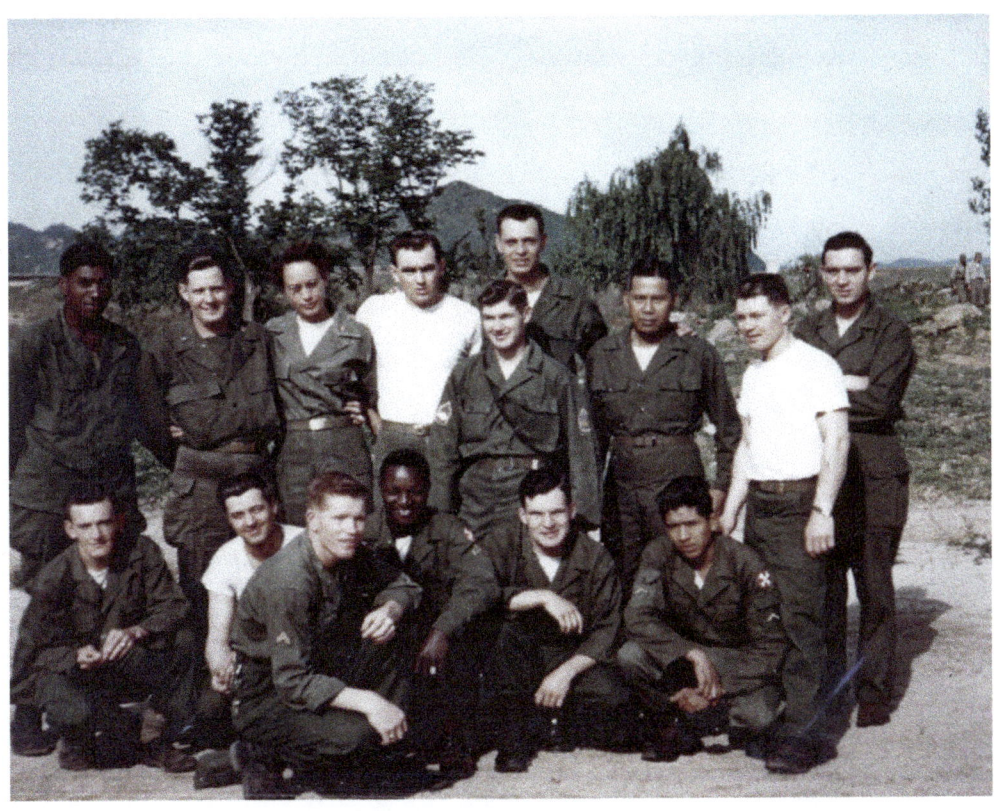

(Photo courtesy of Virginia Taylor collection)

Front L to R:
1. SFC William D. Anderson — Crew Chief
2. CPL Joseph J. Canatella — Cook
3. CPL Selby L. Hawley — Medic/Asst Crew Chief
4. CPL Charles C. Jackson — Medic/Car Commander
5. PFC Mewell H. Tate — Medic/Car Commander
6. CPL Ray W. Costa — Medic/Car Commander

Back L to R:
7. PFC Willie -- McCray — Medic/Car Commander
8. PFC Joseph P. Keevan — Medic/Car Commander
9. 1st Lt. Virginia M. Taylor — Nurse
10. CPL Norton O. Lodahl — Cook
11. PFC Louis O. Mosher — Medic/Car Commander
12. SFC Donald F. Hullopeter — Tech
13. CPL Andrew A. Cadelinia — Warrant Officer
14. SGT Lloyd H. Englebyecht — Mess Sergeant/Cook
15. SGT Kenneth C. Chartier — Tech

(Not pictured: SGT Frederick A. Anderson (Medic), PFC Wilfred L. Bane (Tech), PFC Harold F. Howard (Warrant Officer)

TRAIN 105 COOKS

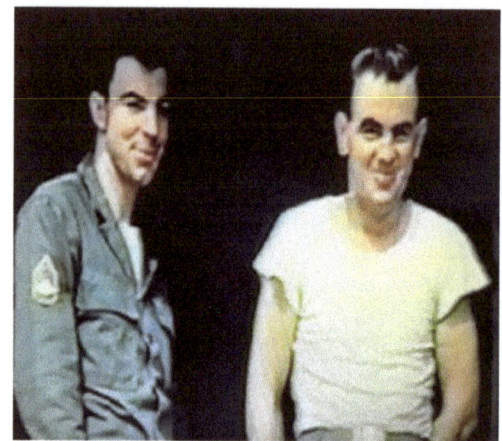

CPLs Joseph Canatella, Norton Lodahl

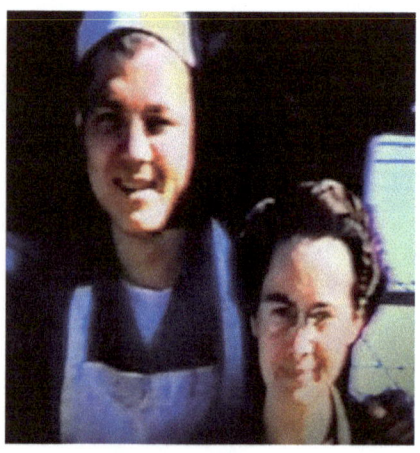

Mess SGT Lloyd Englebyecht (Chief Cook) with Virginia Taylor

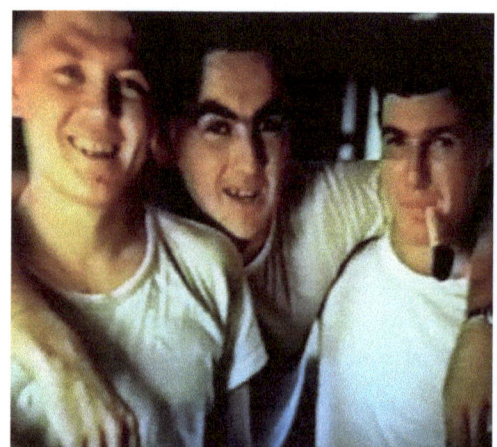

Englebyecht, Lodahl, Canatella

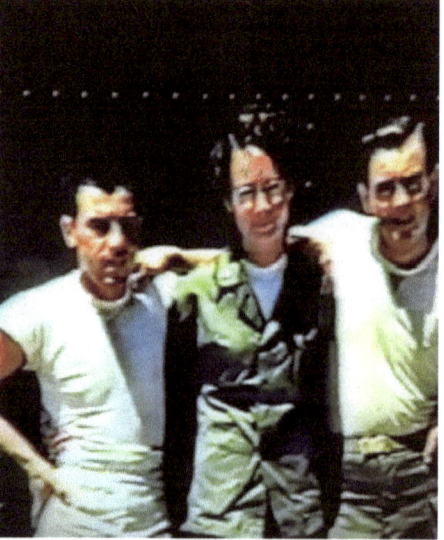

Canatella, Taylor, Lodahl

(Photos courtesy of Virginia Taylor collection)

TRAIN 105 MEDICS

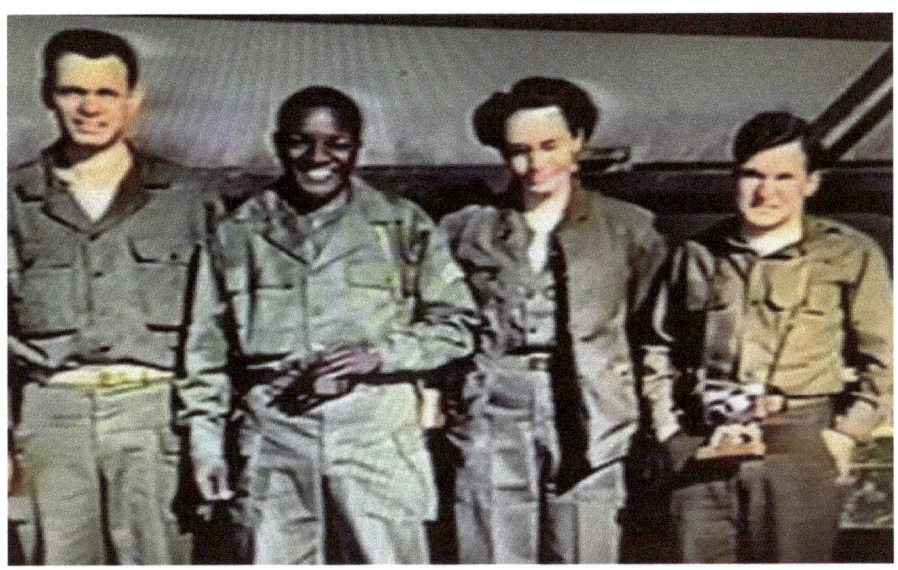

PFC Louis Mosher (Medic)   CPL Charles Jackson (Medic)   Lt. Virginia Taylor (Nurse)   PFC Mewell Tate (Medic)

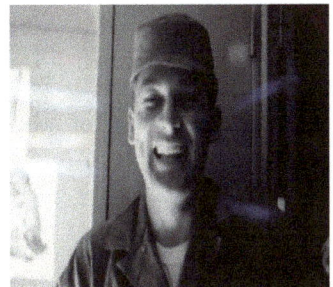

CPL Shelby Hawley (Medic)

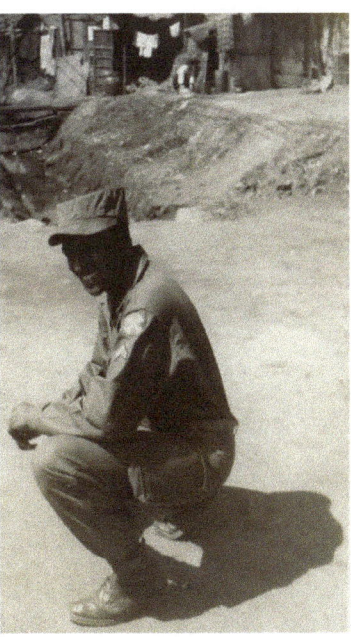

CPL Charles Jackson (Medic)

(Photos courtesy of Virginia Taylor collection)

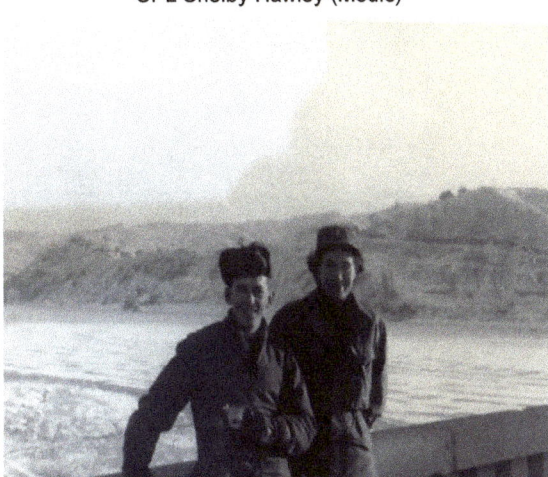

PFC Joseph Keevan (Medic) and Lt. Virginia Taylor (Han River)

DOWNTIME FOR THE CREW (TRAIN 105)

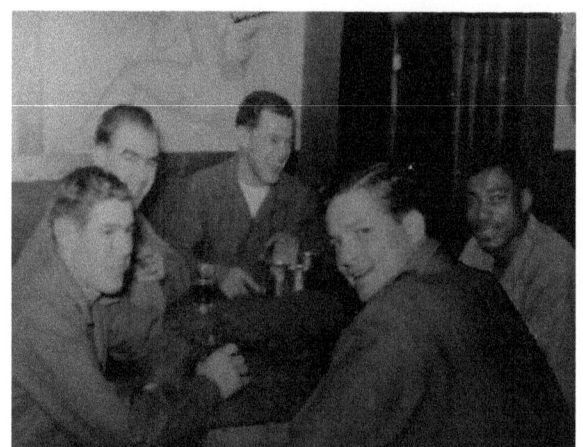

LtoR: Hullopeter, Lodahl, Johnny, McCray (Medic), and Roberts.

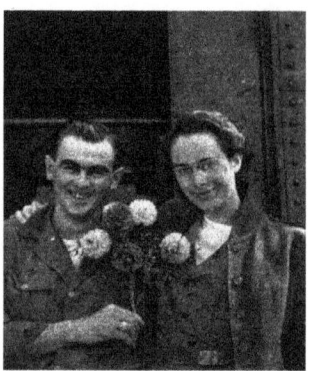

Lodahl and Virginia

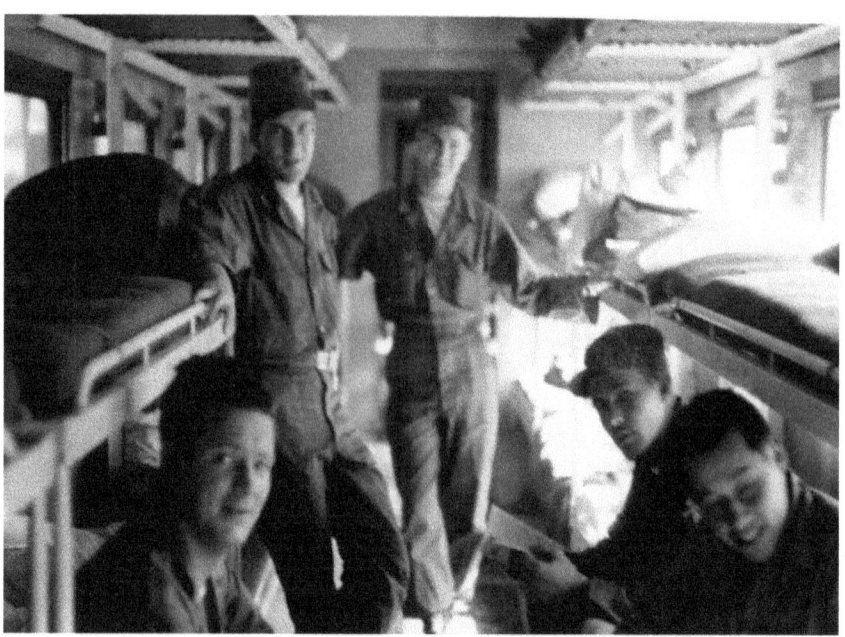

Train 105 Car Commanders (Medics) and crew relax on trip north.
LtoR: Tate, Roberts, Keevan, Hawley, Cadelinia

(Photos courtesy of Virginia Taylor collection)

TRAIN 105 TECH CREW/WARRANT OFFICERS

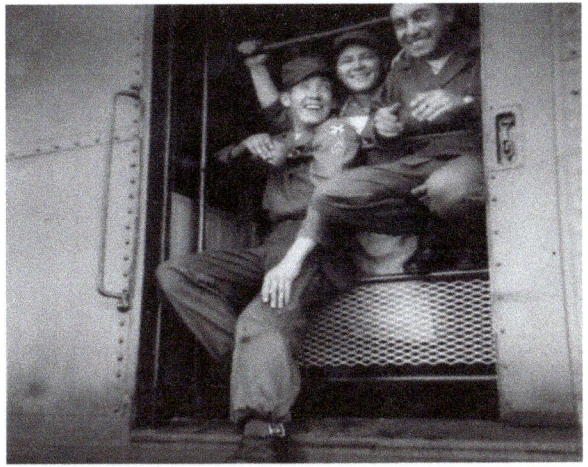

L to R: PFC William J. Eachus, Train Maintenance,
CPL Harry L. Greger MP, SGT Kenneth Chartier, Tech

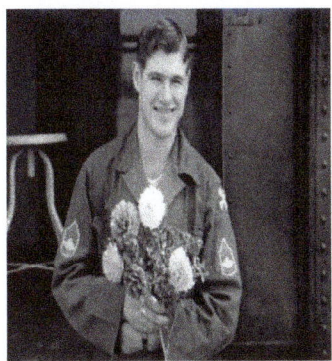

SFC Donald Hullopeter

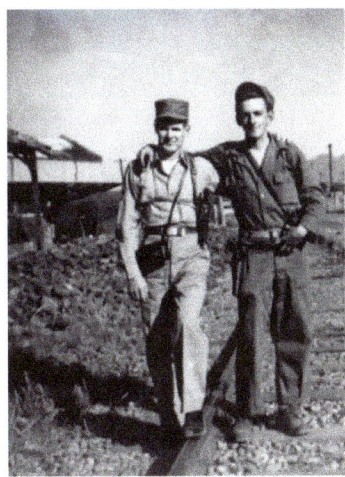

PFCs Harold Howard and Wilfred Bane

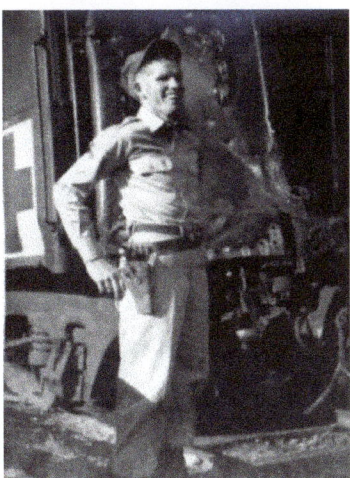

Warrant Officer Train 105
(Photos courtesy of Virginia Taylor)

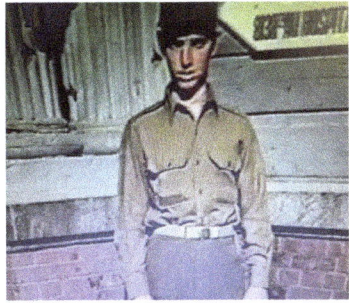

Crew Chief SFC William (Andy) Anderson

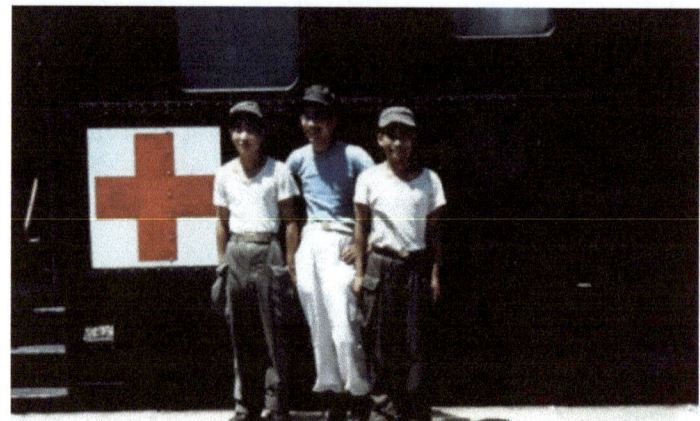

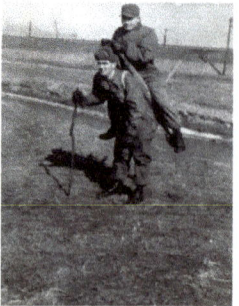

Cooks Lodahl and Englebyecht

Train 105 Korean Helpers

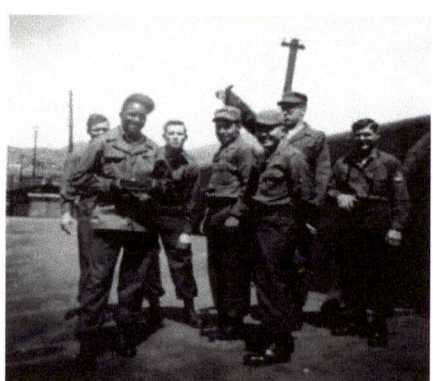

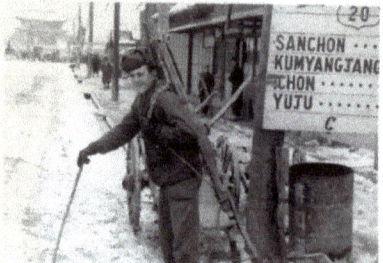

Medic Keevan with Korean A-Frame (SUWON)

Train 105: McCray, Hawley, Costa, Eachus, Hullopeter (PUSAN)

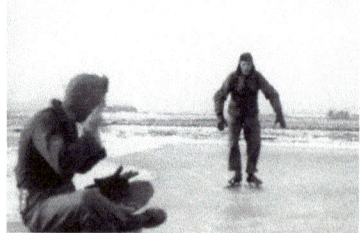

Crew Chief Anderson on ice skates (SUWON)

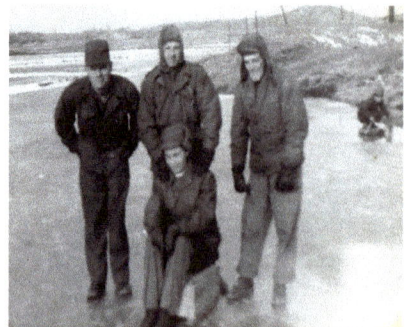

Greger, Chartier, Anderson, Virginia Taylor on box sled sitting on ICE (SUWON)

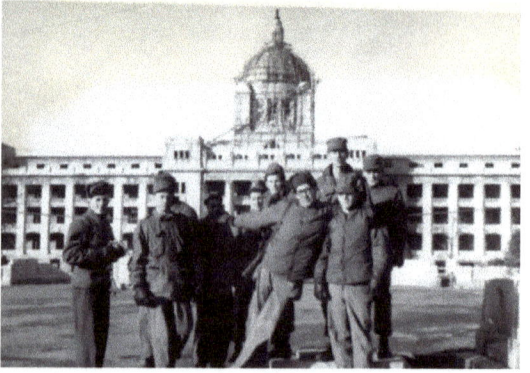

Train 105 Crew at Capital (SEOUL)
LtoR: Keevan, Chartier, Eachus and Greger.
(Photos courtesy of Virginia Taylor collection)

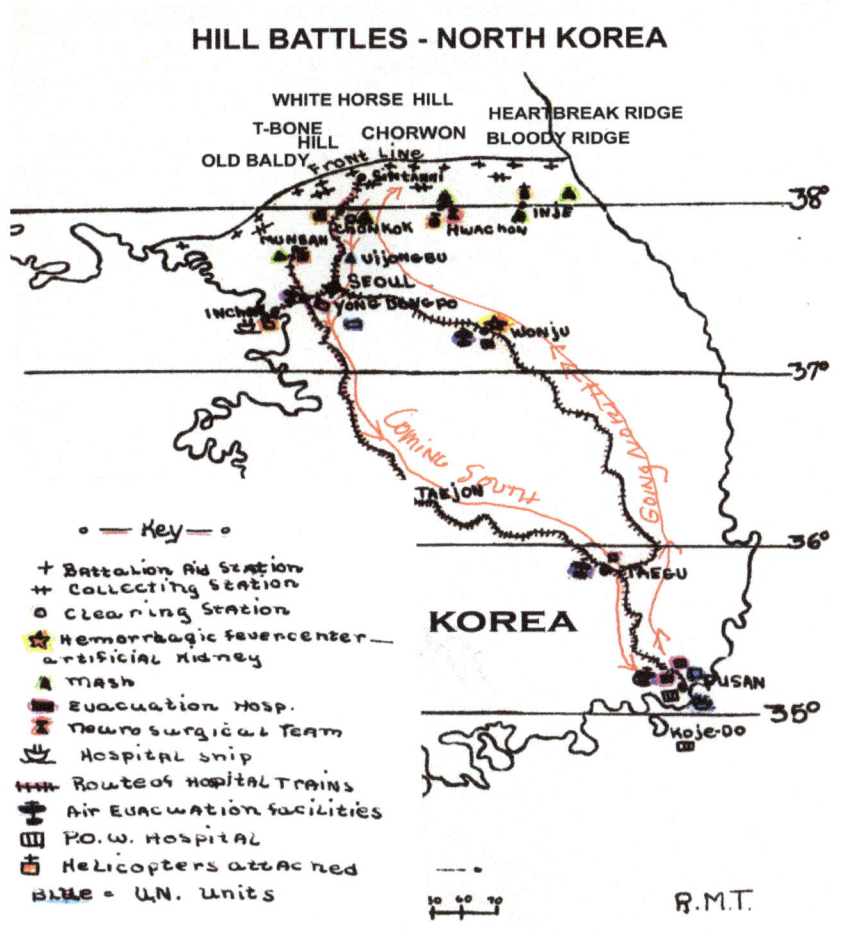

After the breakdown of the Armistice negotiations in August 1951, the UN Command launched a limited offensive to shorten and straighten sections of their lines along the 38th parallel to acquire better defensive terrain and deny the enemy key vantage points to observe and target UN positions.[44] The strategy was to put as much pressure to the other side during negotiations. Bloody Ridge was the first attempt to seize a series of hills. The Chinese and North Korean forces were heavily fortified with reinforced systems. The fighting was intense, mostly with hand-to-hand combat or grenades. By September 5, 1951, the communists were pushed off Bloody Ridge but reestablished a new line 1,500 meters away at what became known as Heartbreak Ridge. Many more hill battles followed into 1953. With repeated Chinese assaults, these hill battles were some of the bloodiest of the war.[45]

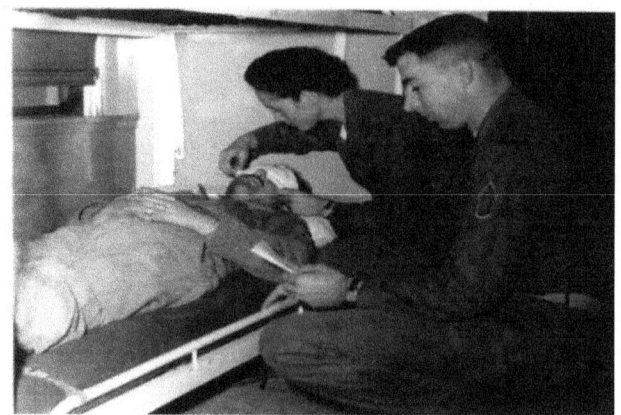

Lt. Virginia Taylor and Crew Chief Andy Anderson tend to a Greek soldier

(Photos courtesy of Virginia Taylor collection)

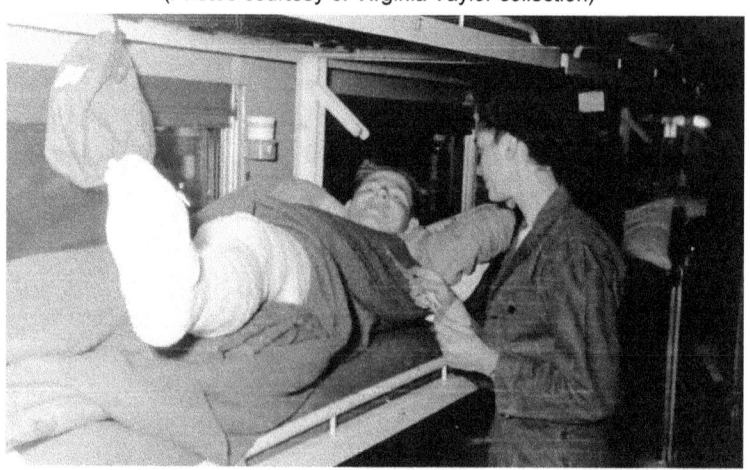

Lt. Virginia Taylor, Nurse Train 105 with patients

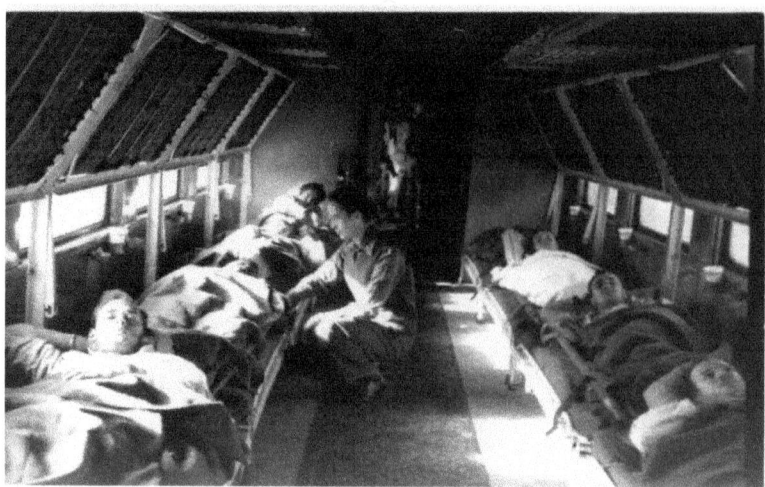

September 1951. Excerpts of Virginia Taylor's letter to her parents:

These colonels and a 2-Star General, General Cross of the 3rd Division, were riding south with us. I gave up my two compartments to two of them and a couple of my corpsmen moved out of theirs. We had 150 patients going south and it kept us hopping.

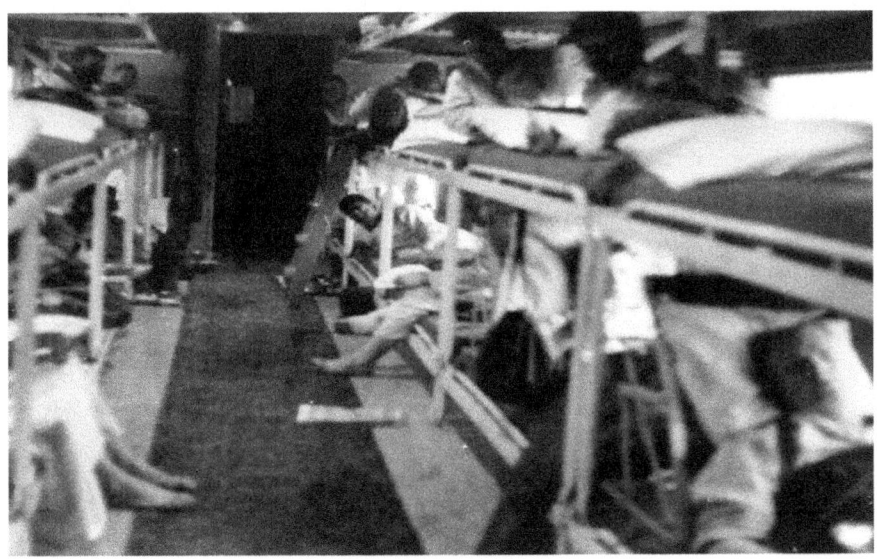

TRAIN 105
(Photo Courtesy of Virginia Taylor collection)

It took 28 hours to get to Pusan and I was so tired with all the extra mess I think I slept 24 hours. On the way down, we met another train going in the opposite direction on the same track. It was just getting dusk. It was lucky as had it been dark, we'd of hit HEAD-ON as we travel at night <u>blacked out</u>—no headlight of any kind. Someone had gotten mixed up with the switches. Koreans run the operations. I guess someone misunderstood an order. Being as Hospital Trains have a No 1 priority when patients aboard, the other train had to back up to the nearest siding about 10 miles. Near Taegu a freight train <u>had been derailed by a bridge being blown up</u>, and the tracks were littered with a big mess which delayed us 2 hours.

The enemy was indifferent to the Western etiquette of war. Attacks on medical personnel, vehicles, and tents became the rule rather than exception. The enemy riflemen used the red crosses on regimental ambulances as bull's eyes. A hospital train leaving Taegu for Pusan was hit by fire from rifles or automatic weapons; later emerging from a tunnel, it was again a target, this time for rifle fire and grenades. As a result, hospital trains had to run in daylight hours, and emergency night runs were guarded by military policemen riding on sandbagged flatcars.[46]

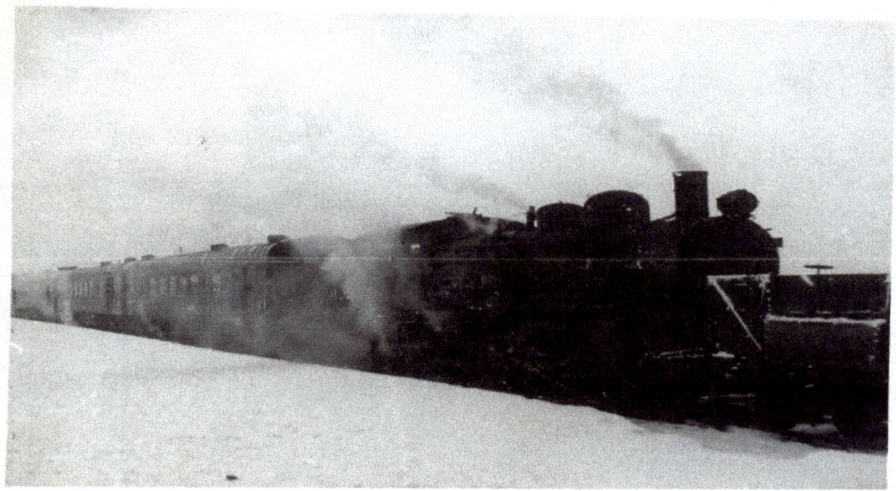

TRAIN 105—Gondola flatcar in front of the engine for the military police.
(Photo courtesy Virginia Taylor collection)

Each train operated with two guard cars, one ahead of the engine and one behind the train. The cars were gondolas with about two feet of sandbags around the inside and level with the top of the car. The sandbags through the middle of the car made two pockets and mounted on each were .30 or .50 caliber machine guns. It was a miserable assignment.[47]

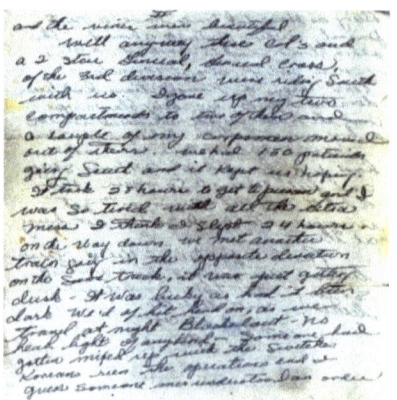

December 23-25, 1951. Excerpts of Virginia Taylor's letter to her parents:

Tomorrow will be Christmas Eve and it hardly seems it to me. We will have a big dinner Christmas day and probably be loading up for our return to Pusan. In spite of it being not like most Christmases we've known—we have a lot to be thankful for—just in the four months that have passed I have given thanks many, many times for I am who I am, not a permanent part of this miserable land.

<u>24 December 51</u>
Sometime during the night, we moved up to Yongdongpo on the outskirts of Seoul. Ice has frozen over all rice paddies and the ground is white with frost. We left No 108 and <u>Captain Toole gang</u> at Suwon.

Capt. Lena Toole (Train 108)

<u>Betty's train 103</u> was at Yongdongpo. When we pulled in could only wave and shout greetings as we passed. She was loaded with casualties and headed for Pusan.

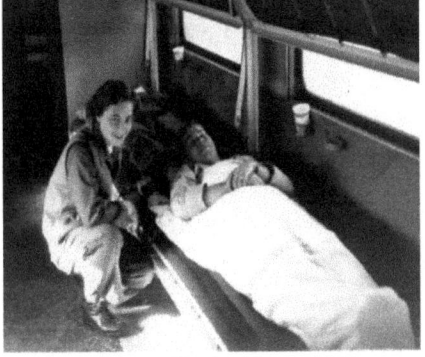

Lt. Betty Potocik (Train 103)
(Photos courtesy of Virginia Taylor collection)

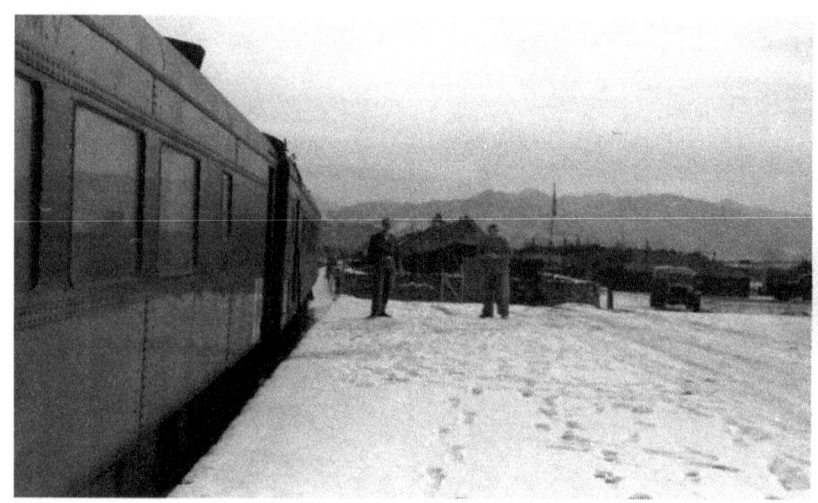

CHONKOK Collecting Station (10 miles above 38th parallel). Tents in background. (Photos courtesy of Virginia Taylor collection)

25 December 51 (Christmas) 7:30 p.m.

We pulled out of Yongdongpo at 0220. Everyone got up for an early breakfast at 0500. At 0700 we stopped at Chonkok, 10 miles North of the 38th. Have an all-tent hospital lay scattered on the cold white ground.

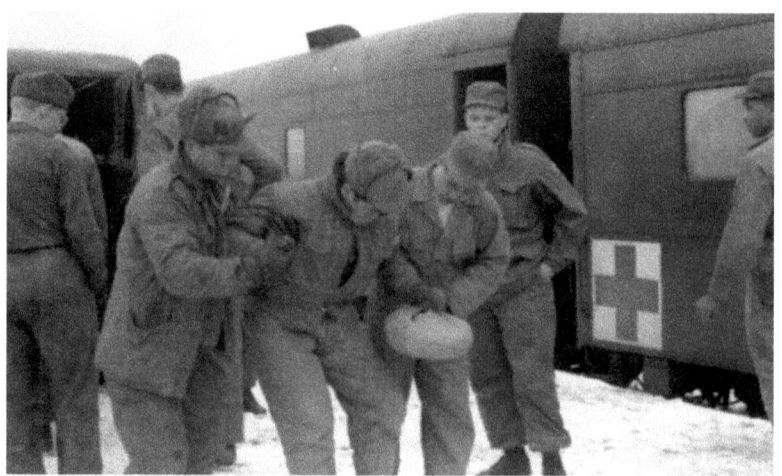

Train 105 Medics Willie McCray and Ray Costa helping MASH patient to the train

At 0800 the ambulances from the Mobile Surgical Units (MASH) began to arrive. The constant thunder of the big guns echoed throughout the valley while we loaded carload after carload of wounded.

December 23-25, 1951. Virginia Taylor's letter (continued):

It gave us all satisfaction and pride as we loaded the dirty tired men into our fresh-clean hospital coaches. **Some had forgotten it was Christmas until they saw our Christmas decorations. Crew Chief— Sgt Anderson of Tennessee—played Santa Claus and passed out our Christmas socks. The cooks had stayed up all night preparing turkey dressing and all that goes with a Christmas menu.** *We left Chonkok at 11 a.m. and got the green light through Yongdongpo. When we started to unload, we were greeted by Col Page, Chief Surgeon of the Far East. Press photographers were snapping bulbs all over the place. I got a lot of good pictures, but it was snowing and kinda dark. I hope they turn out.*

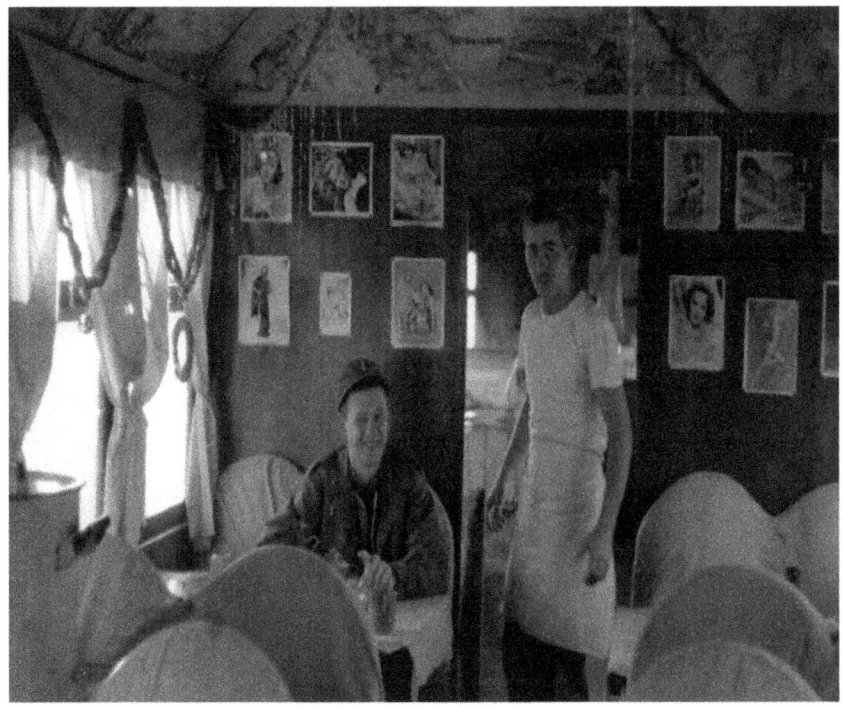

Train 105 Kitchen/Dining Car decorated with Christmas chains, wreaths, and balls on the curtains. Icicles hung from the roof. Nurse Virginia Taylor made the curtains.

(Photo courtesy of Virginia Taylor collection)

III

Tomorrow will be Christmas eve and it hardly seems it to me. We will have a big dinner Christmas day and probably be loading up for our return to Pusan. In spite of it being not like most Christmases we've known — we have a lot to be thankful for — Just in the four months that have passed I have given thanks many many times that I am who I am and not a permanent part of this miserable land.

0815
24 Dec 1951

Sometime during the night we moved up to Yong dong po on the outskirts of Seoul. Ice has frozen over all the rice paddies and the ground is white with frost. We left no 108 & Capt Tooles gang at Suwon. Betty's train, 103, was at Yong dong po when we pulled in. Could only wave & shout greetings as we passed. She was loaded with casualties & headed for Pusan.

1945 (730 pm)
25 Dec.
Christmas.

We pulled out of Yong dong po @ 0220. Everyone got up for an early breakfast @ 0500.

At 0700 we stopped at Chum chon — or Chonbok, 10 miles north of the 38th. Here an all tent Hospital lay scattered on the cold white ground. At 0800 the ambulances from the mobile surgical units began to arrive — the constant thunder of the big guns echoed throughout the valley while we loaded carload after carload of wounded. It gave us all satisfaction and pride as we loaded the dirty tired men into our fresh clean Hospital coaches. Some had forgotten it was Christmas until they saw our Christmas decorations. Crew Chief Sgt Anderson of Tennessee played Santa Claus and passed out our Christmas Socks. The cooks had stayed up all night preparing turkey, dressing and all that goes with a Christmas menu. We left Chonbok at 11 AM and got the green light through to Yong dong po. When we started to unload we were greeted by Col Page Chief Surgeon of the Far East — Press photographers were snapping bulbs all over the place. I got a lot of good pictures — but it was snowing & kinda dark I hope they turn out.

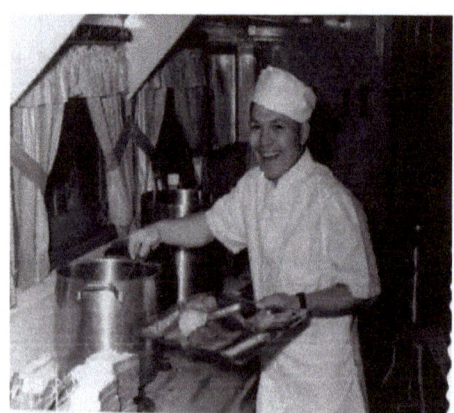

Lloyd Englebyecht
Mess Sgt/Chief Cook Train 105

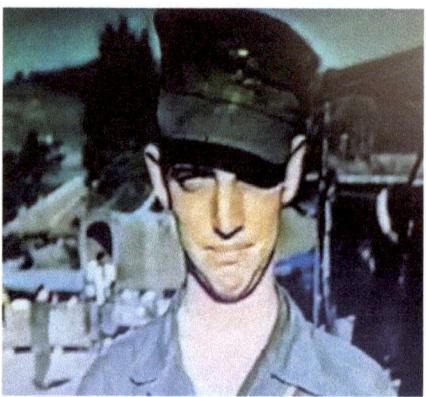

Crew Chief Andy Anderson dressed as Santa Claus to hand out Christmas stockings to the wounded.

(Photos courtesy of Virginia Taylor collection)

January 30, 1952. Excerpts of Virginia Taylor's letter to her parents:

Things are pretty quiet here. Had only 133 patients on the last load; 30 were frostbites from the severe cold. One boy was wounded in his upper legs and <u>had to drag himself for a day and a-half</u> to an aid station for help as his outfit had withdrawn and somehow he had got cut off from the line. His feet and hands were in terrible shape, having damage of the deep tissues. "It was a miracle he found friendly lines again," he says and continually thanked God that he was alive.

We have special frostbite solution mixed with Heparin (an anti coagulant drug) which picks up circulation to the affected area, which is given all frostbite cases of 6 hours intravenously. So before we got to Taegu, the frostbite center, we had given 90 bottles of the stuff in the men's veins.

Men pinned down in the snow or isolated by enveloping attacks were in no position to prevent frostbite. Peaks in cold injury coincided with peaks in enemy activity. Besides the severe weather, many times below zero, the prescribed footwear—the shoepack, a winterized boot worn over heavy socks and felt insoles added to the problem. A cycle often set up of perspiration, maceration, and the development of so-called shoepac foot followed by hospitalization for 10 to 15 days became a repeated cycle. Troops were urged to remove the boot frequently and dry the socks and insole. Not a realistic solution under battlefield conditions.[48] Severe cases of frostbite, as described above, mummified the extremities, forced amputation, and required months of treatment.

Virginia Taylor's February 25, 1952 letter to her parents provided an update on the above patient: *The frostbite (patient) you asked about was flown to Japan several days ago and was expected to lose only his toes.*

February 25, 1952, Pusan 21st Evac Hospital. Excerpts of Virginia Taylor's letter to her parents:

It's storming up a gale outside, dreary and cold. Our little ole pot belly is glowing cheerfully, making things cozy and warm in the big room.

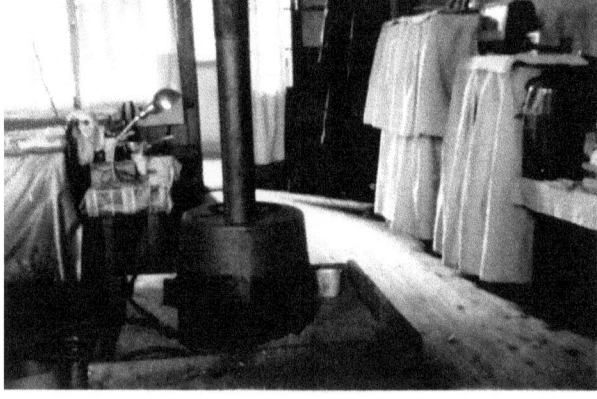

Virginia Taylor's quarters at the 21st EVAC Hospital
Potbelly stove

Virginia shared these quarters with three nurses:
Betty, Sal, and Nickey

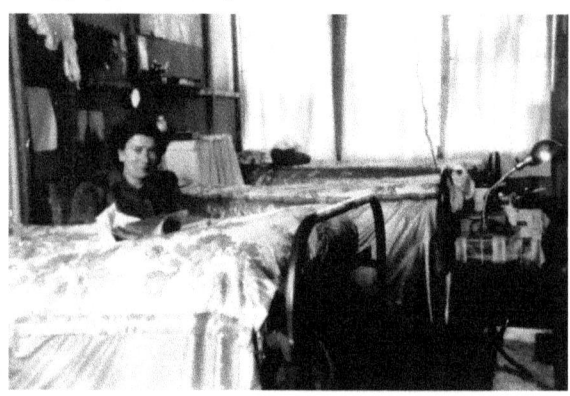

Roommate Betty Potocik (Train 103)

I got back from the north run on Friday, being only a 3-1/2 day trip we had it easy going. One of my patients, Cpl Alxander of the 45th Inf. Division (Thunderbirds) from the Oklahoma National Guard was due to rotate soon and was going to stop and visit relatives who lived in Alameda, so I wrote a note to Rosie and he is going to drop in and say hello. (Rosie was Virginia's sister.)

February 25, 1952. Excerpts of Virginia Taylor's letter to parents (continued):

The actual battle casualties have been light on the west front and our main concern at present is the frostbite, pneumonias and Hemorrhagic Fever. The frostbite (patient) you asked about was flown to Japan several days ago and was expected to lose only his toes.

On Saturday a group of us visited the Chishoms and stayed for the evening service. The little group has grown—many servicemen, officers and UN troops—now attend the meetings.

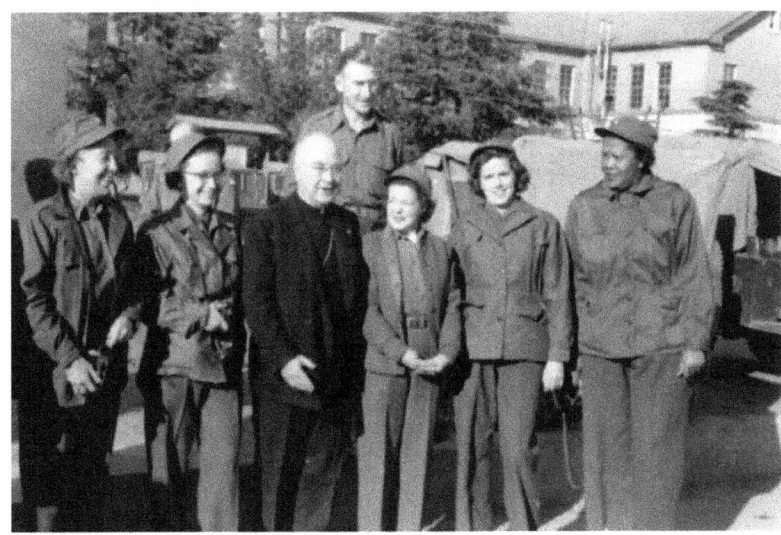

(Photo courtesy of Virginia Taylor collection)

I have bought me a 35mm camera, which takes color slide pictures as well as black and whites. Will send a viewer and my boxes of slides as I take them and you will get a better picture of what the place is really like.

Am sending a couple clippings—one a write up of Seoul which I thought was a good description. One is of the Freedom Bridge where our HOSPITAL TRAINS will cross, if and when, the Panmunjom Peace is settled.

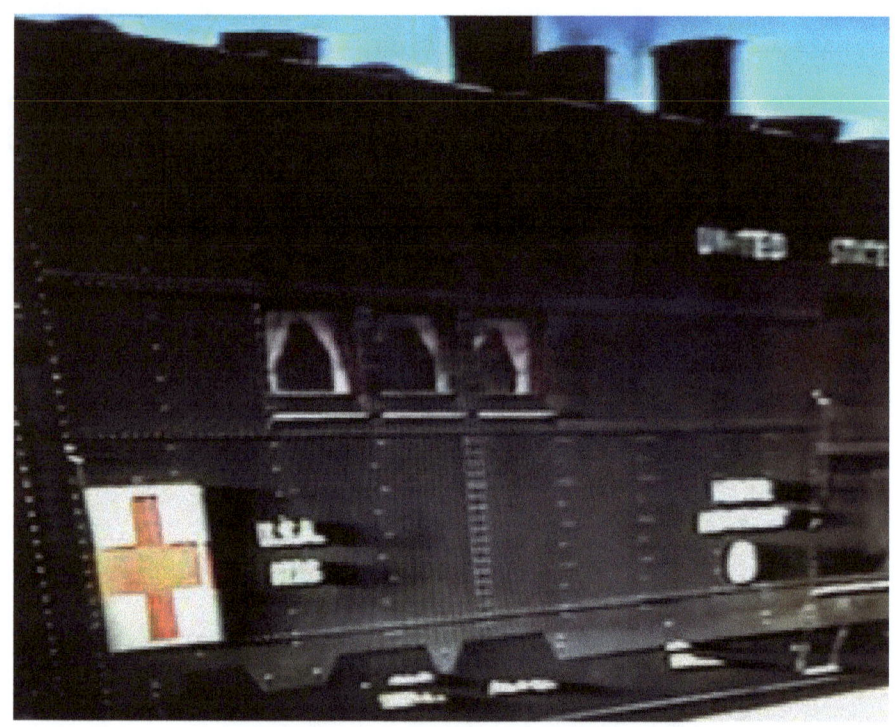

Virginia's curtains viewed from the outside
Train 105 Kitchen Car

(Photo courtesy of Virginia Taylor collection)

Have ordered from Sears some plastic material for curtains for our kitchen car. A lot of rivalry exists amongst the trains—each crew thinks they have the best train and everyone tries to outdo the other. TRAIN 105 is the best though (heh).

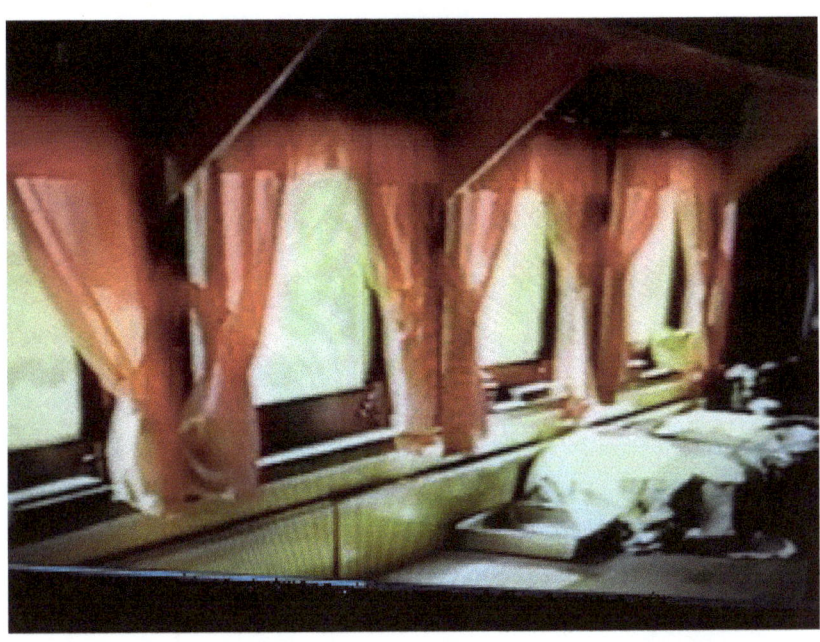

Red curtains made by Virginia Taylor for the Kitchen/Dining car Train 105

June 16, 1952, Excerpts of Virginia Taylor's letter to parents:

Since the last I wrote, on June 2, we've made 2 trips to the front and back. A lot of heavy fighting around Chorwon by the 45th Division has given us some heavy loads.

Am now at the 21st Evac in Pusan and expect to head NORTH at six p.m. It is Father's Day today, and as usual, I'm the cows tail again, always late. It is sort of a dark dreary day and everyone is sitting about reading or sleeping.

Last week we got a package from the Pennsylvania RR with our XYLOPHONE in it—<u>each week we add something new to the train keeping us way out in front of the others.</u>

Virginia and her crew were in competition with the other trains to make Train 105 the BEST. (Reference letter written to her parents February 25, 1952—red curtains for the dining car.) *As much as it was a competition, they wanted to add extra touches for the wounded soldiers to give them a little piece of home.* Before dinner was served, the kitchen helper would walk from car to car playing the Xylophone, same as they did on the Pennsylvania RR back home. Each bar produced a different **pitch**: the shorter the bar, the higher the **pitch**. He would tap four bars, starting with the **lower pitch first**.

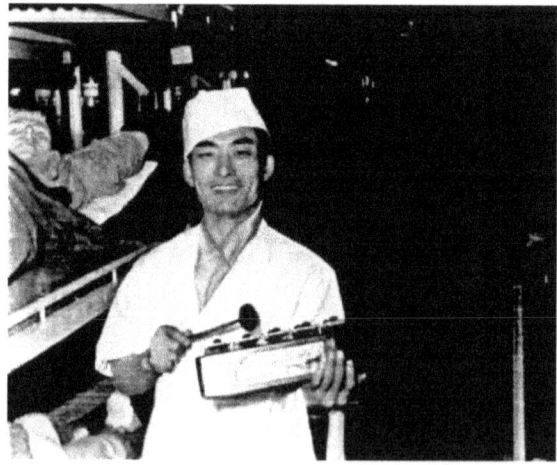

49

(Photo courtesy by Virginia Taylor collection)

JARED INGERSOLL
GIRARD TRUST BUILDING
PHILADELPHIA 2, PA.

May 8, 1952

Lt. Virginia M. Taylor
Hospital Train #105
A.P.O. 301
c/o Post Master

Dear Lieutenant:

I have your letter of April 25, which has just been received, and I appreciate very much receiving it.

I immediately got in touch with the Pennsylvania Railroad, and they are sending you direct a xylophone, which I sincerely hope may be of some help to you in your fine work, and I hope it is received soon.

I am also taking the liberty of enclosing a $20 bill, which I hope you can personally use in any way you think might be helpful to the morale of your group.

With best of luck in what you are doing, which many of us here in this country are deeply appreciative of, I remain

Very sincerely yours,

C. Jared Ingersoll

CJI:FPG
Enclosure
AIR MAIL

Sgt. Anderson, my crew chief, went home on emergency leave last week. He wrote that his wife was out of danger and that he would be back to Korea in a month. We miss him, but it's a shame he has to come back. (Sgt. Anderson played Santa Claus on the train—reference letter December 1951.)

Have had a cold for past week or so, so haven't ventured out. With the heat of summer, the filth and dust and fleas seem to increase. What a miserable land.

June 25, 1952. Excerpts of Virginia Taylor's letter to her sister (Rosie):

Today we loaded up north again with casualties of the 45th Inf. Division (Oklahoma National Guard) wounded in the battle for what they call "Shanghi Heights" near Chorwon. At present time we are clicking along some where between Taejon and Taegu and most of the patients are alseep. In the past week or so we've been meeting ourselves coming and going. Today being the 2-year anniversary of the war, another big push is expected. I wish this whole mess was over with.

It has been terrible hot here the past week and we stay in our air-conditioned areas most of the time. It is a blessing to have it cool for the wounded. I guess we are the only ones who have ice and cool quarters in Korea. The Army gives to its wounded the best medical care in the world.

It's sort of interesting to watch the changes in the rice fields on each trip up. First we see the small green tufts for miles and miles. Next trip, they will be new plants—then a whole sea of beautiful deep green.

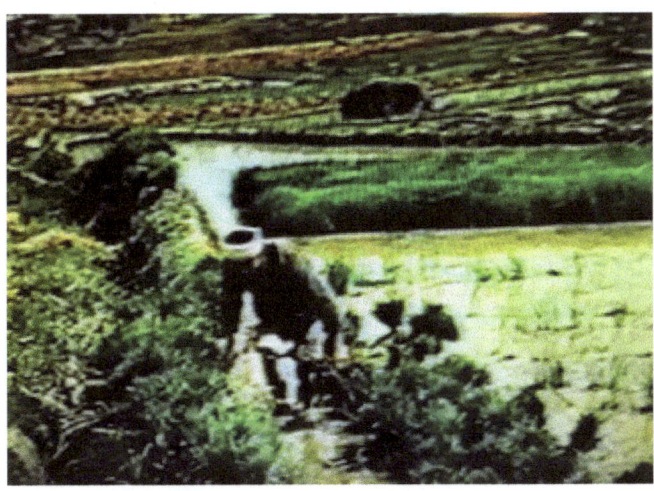

Worker in rice paddy
(Photo courtesy of Virginia Taylor collection)

Then the harvest, and now just the dried up tufts left after the harvest. Next week old Papasan will have his oxen and wooden plow—replowing and irrigating for his second crop of the season.

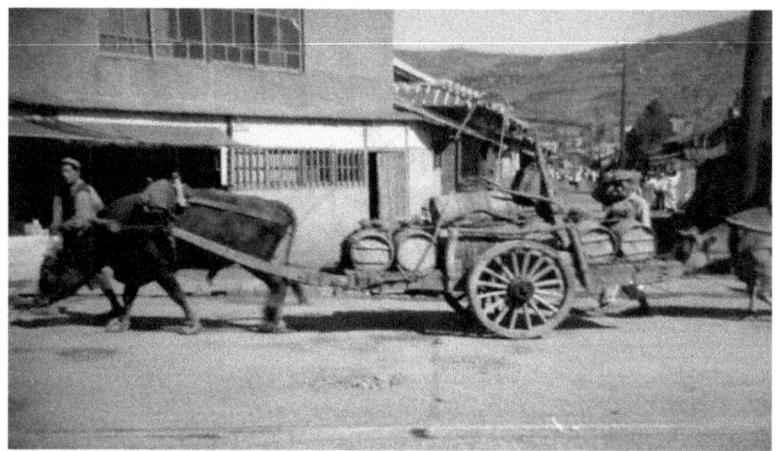

(Photos courtesy of Virginia Taylor collection)

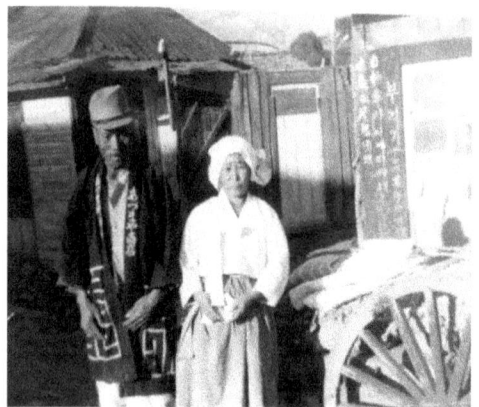

Papasan and Mamasan in their Sunday best

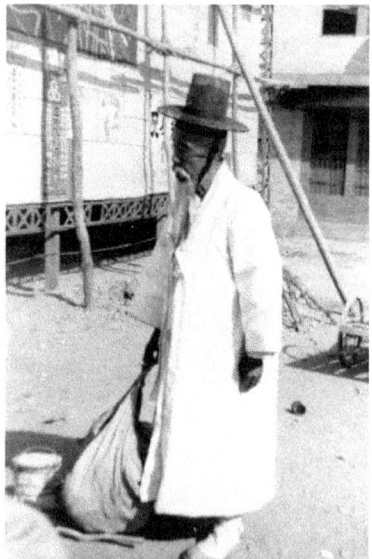

Old, Old Papasan

In every available piece of land something is planted. Nothing is wasted. Many people are homeless and hundreds die of starvation and malnutrition. The land and cities are twisted and torn. Filth, flies, dust, and misery predominate. <u>I thank myself a million times a day that I am an American.</u>

July 24, 1952 excerpts, Yongdongpo, Korea. Excerpts of Virginia Taylor's letter to her parents:

At the present time we are sitting on a side track waiting for clearance on a northbound track. For the past 10 days we've been running our heads off with casualties from the 2nd Infantry Division in the battle for "Old Mt Baldy." It is hotter than the shades of Hell and that's just putting it mildly. Sometimes we have ice for our air conditioning bunkers and sometimes we don't. The coaches are sometimes 110-120 degrees. I and the crew and the patients are exhausted after the long run to Pusan. Boy! My Kingdom for a shade tree and a mountain stream and a big strawberry soda.

July 26, 1952 (midnight)

Now about 3 hours out of Taejon headed south with only 150, it rained today and we got ice for the bunkers so it's been a comfortable trip for most everyone. Seems like I write about the same thing each time, but there just isn't anything much to say. The days are pretty much routine as are the weeks and months. Head north for Chonkok, load up with patients, come south with patients, stay in Pusan 3 or 4 days and head north again for another load of wounded battle-weary men.

TODAY the train stopped along side of an 18-coach troop train loaded with about 500 fresh troops headed for the 2nd Div area near Chorwon and old "Mt Baldy" and "T-Bone Ridge." One could read the thoughts of every man on the troop train as he looked across at the wounded on the Hospital Train. **Most of them were young kids.** *No one smiled or joked. They all looked grim, and worried, and old.*

Thoughts were running through my mind too of how many of those fellows would make the return trip home and who would be riding the Hospital Train on the next trip.

One soldier yelled across asking where we'd come from. We answered, "Near the front." We asked where they were headed. He answered, "The FRONT." That's all anybody said. Both train loads of men stared at each other in silence until the trains pulled away.

IT'S A HELL of a war is all I can say. I wonder when someone is going to wake up to the fact that men are still dying here. Somebody's son isn't going to come home.

1952 summer monsoons and autumnal heavy rains turned the **battle terrains** above MUNSAN—**Old Baldy, Siberia Heights, and Bunker Hill**—into six-inch deep mud. Bunkers caved in, bridges washed out, and roads were several feet under water. The division surgeon called upon the Navy for the amphibious DUKWs to carry in supplies to the flooded areas and to bring out the wounded.[50] The wounded Marines were transported to the Marine Division Clearing Station in Munsan. When the hospital train arrived, they were transported again to the train by DUWKs.

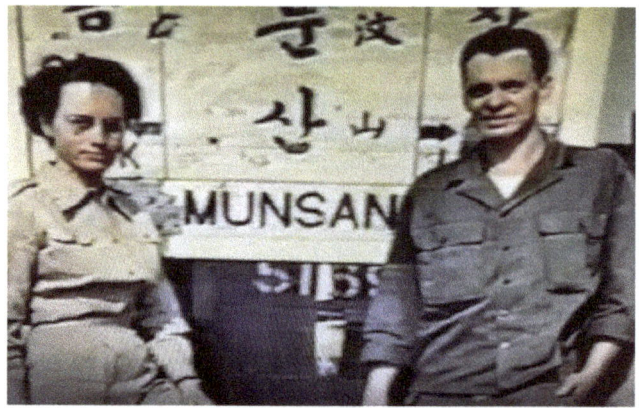

Nurse 1st Lt. Virginia Taylor and Medic PFC Louis Mosher
MUNSAN, Korea, Marine Division Clearing Station

(Photos courtesy Virginia Taylor collection)

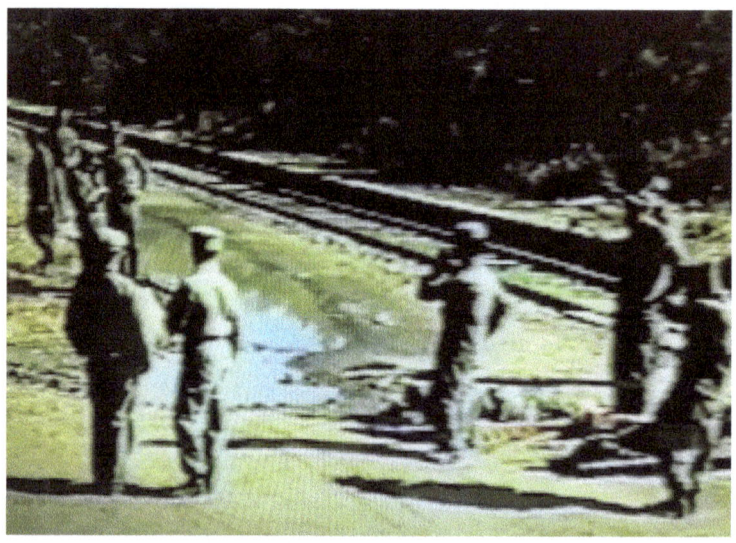

Muddy Terrain

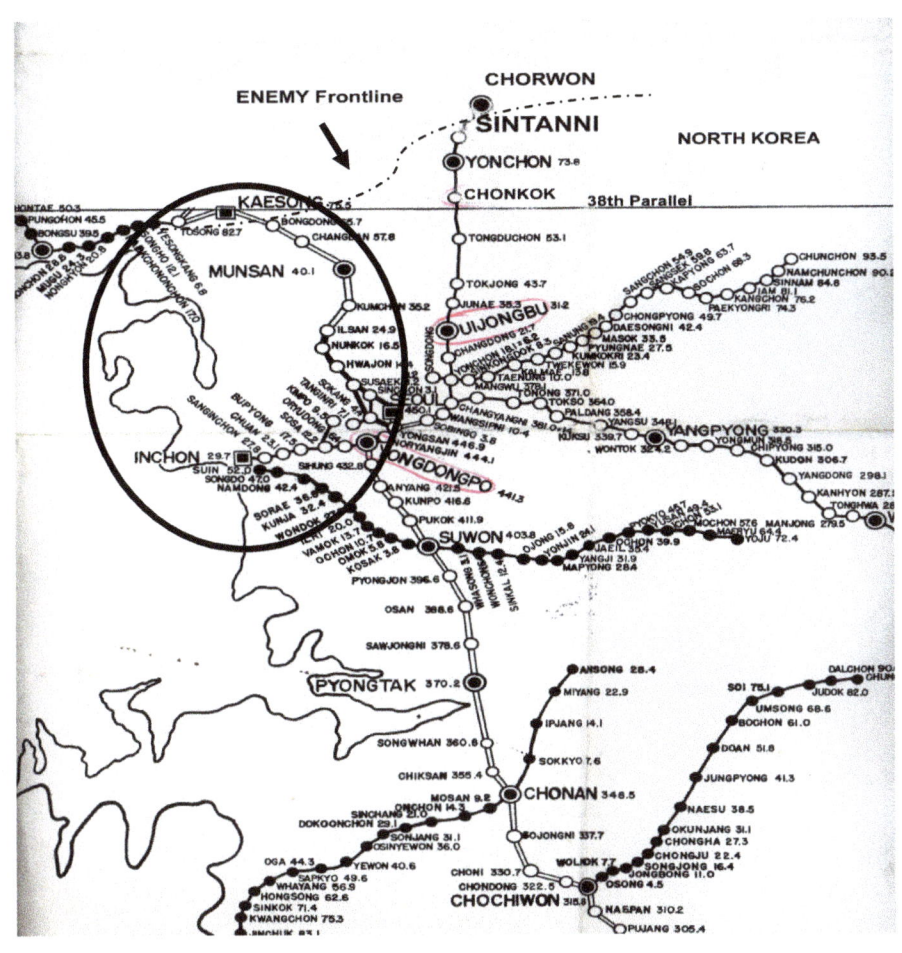

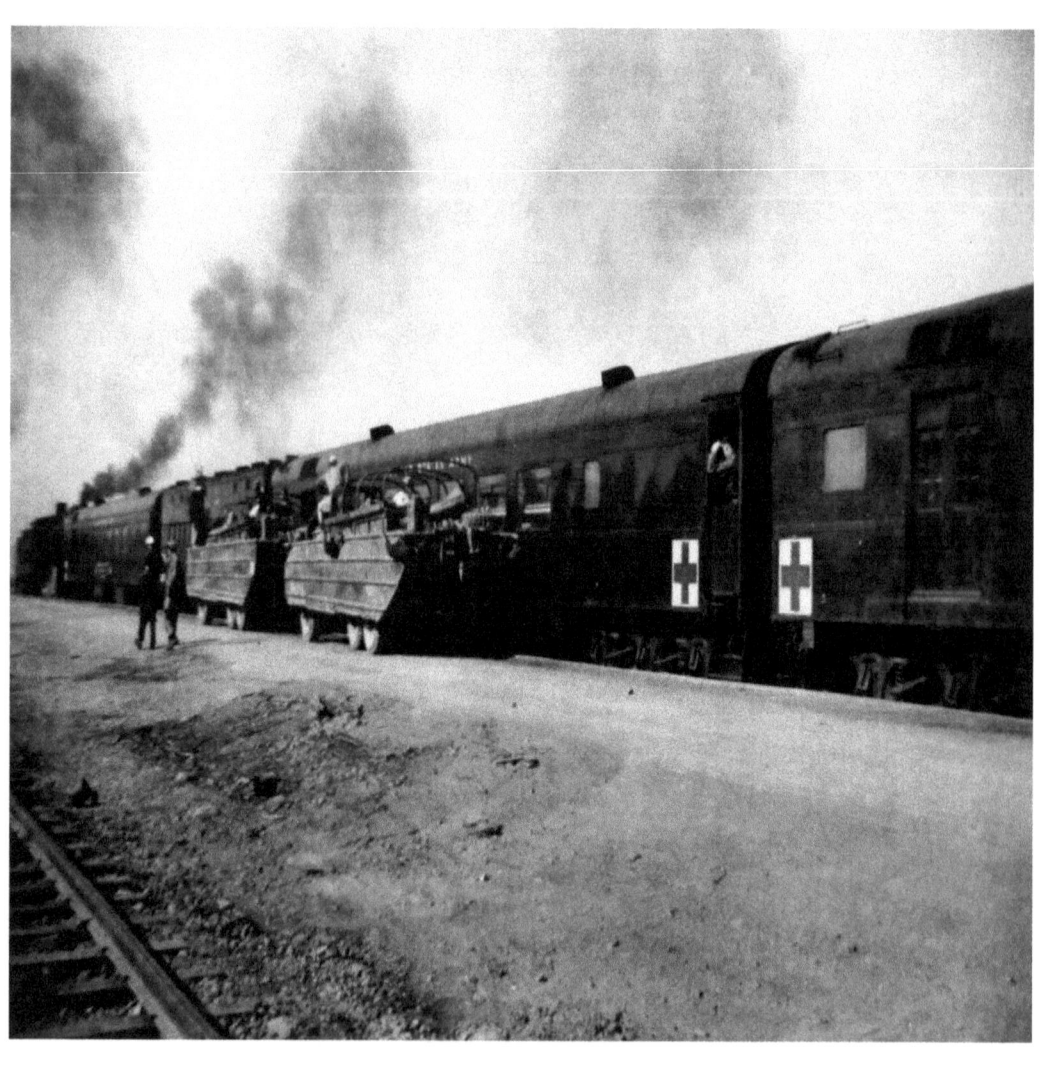

MUNSAN, Korea (Marine Div Clearing Station)
Wounded Marines brought to Train 105 by DUKWs

(Photo courtesy of Virginia Taylor collection)

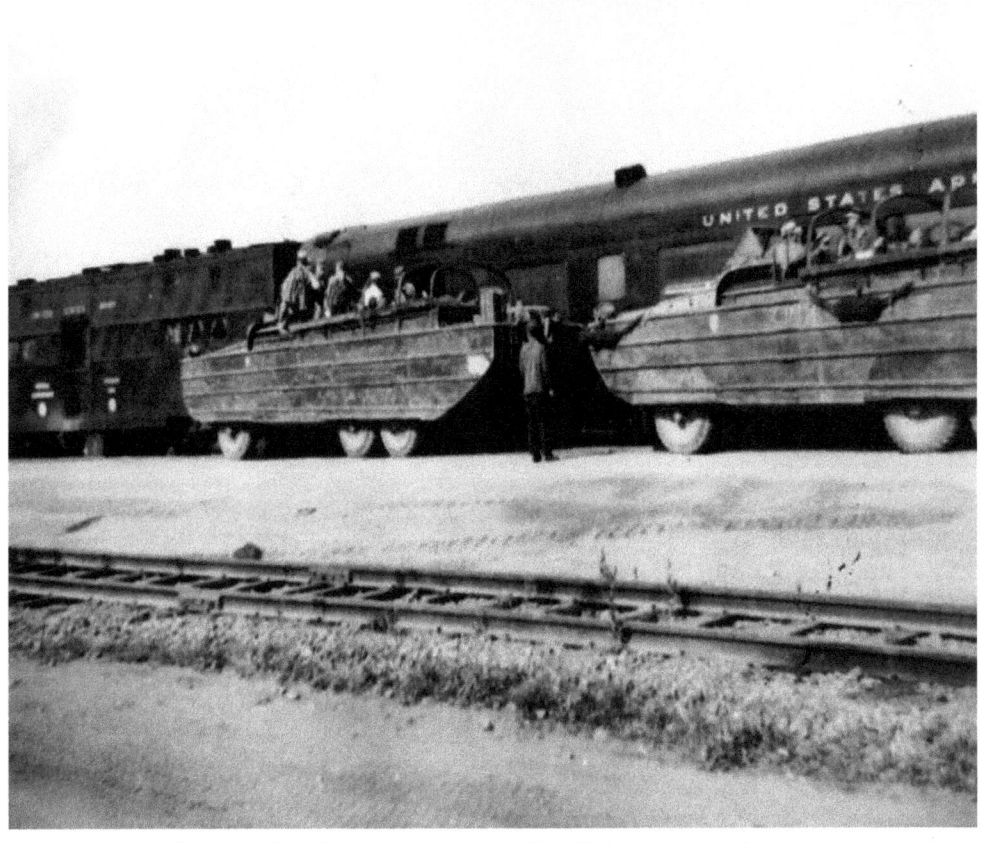

Note Virginia Taylor's curtains in the kitchen-car windows

(Photo courtesy of Virginia Taylor collection)

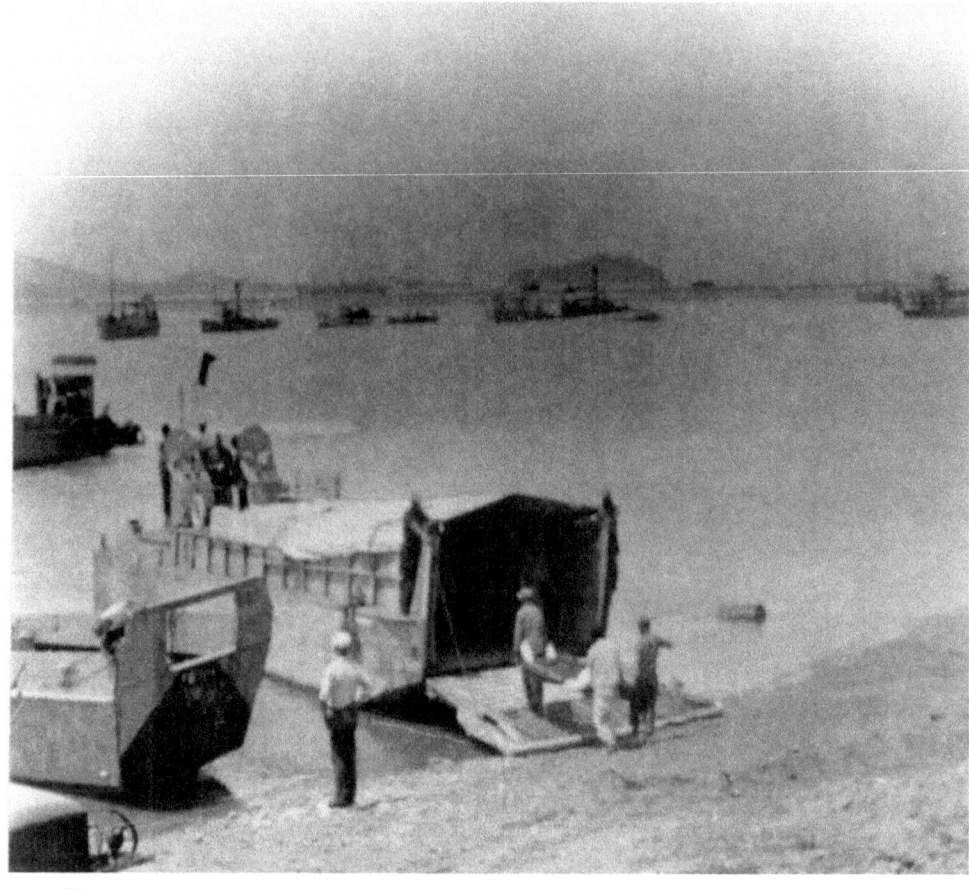
The train brought the wounded Marines from Munsan to INCHON HARBOR. There, they were loaded onto a LST for transport to the Navy hospital ship anchored out in the bay.

(Photo courtesy of Virginia Taylor's collection)

August 19, 1952, 21st Evac Hospital, Pusan. Excerpts of Virginia Taylor's letter to her parents:

It is a cool quiet evening here in Pusan, a little rain now and then settling the dust, and a good ocean breeze, giving some fresh clean air.

Returned yesterday from the North. **Loaded at Munsan with many Marines from the fierce battle 7 miles north of Munsan on a place designated as "Siberian Heights" and "Bunker Hill."** *It seems like such a useless waste of life to take a hill, then lose it, then recapture it and lose it again. Many lives lost and nothing gained.*

I have bought a movie camera 16mm Kodak so will bring home movies of all this going on. Have many color slides to show, also taken on my Nikon Japanese Camera with 1:4 lens.

TOMORROW at 1300 the HOSPITAL TRAIN UNIT is being presented with a <u>Presidental Unit Citation</u> down at the pier. We all have to stand formation. Eight nurses, 6 doctors, 120 corpsman, and 25 men from the maintenance section will get the award. <u>We all think it's pretty wonderful</u>. Some of my friends from the 21st Evac Hospital are going down and taking pictures, so will get some movies too.

A huge General ship came into Pusan Harbor today and unloaded with 4,000 fresh troops. They were marched directly off the gang plank onto 5 or 6 troop trains and are now headed North. I have been thinking of them and what they must be thinking tomorrow evening. They'll be up front fighting and dodging shrapnel. Yesterday they were drinking cokes.

19 Aug 52
Tuesday
2137 Hrs

Dearest Folks,

It is a cool quiet evening here in Pusan, a little rain: now & then settling the dust, and a good ocean breeze, giving some fresh clear air.

Returned yesterday from the north. Loaded at Munsan with many marines from the fierce battle 7 miles north of Munsan on a place designated as "Siberia Heights" and "Bunker Hill." It seems like such a useless waste of life. To take a hill, then loose it, then recapture it & loose it again — many lifes lost & nothing gained.

I have bought a movie camera 16 mm Kodak so will bring home movies of all this goings on. Have many color slides to show also taken on my Nikon Japanese Camera with 1.4 lens.

Tomorrow at 1300 the Hospital Train Unit is being presented with a Presidential Unit Citation down at the pier. We all have to stand Formation. 8 nurses, 6 Doctors, 120 corpsman and 25 men from the maintance section will get the award. We all think its pretty wonderful. Some of my friends from the 21st are going down & take pictures so will get some movies too.

A huge General ship came into Pusan harbor today & unloaded with 4000 fresh troops. They were marched directly off the gang plank onto 5 or 6 troop trains and one now headed North. I have been thinking of them and what they must be thinking. Tomorrow evening they'll be up front fighting & dodging shapnel. Yesterday they were drinkin' cokes

September 9, 1952 (Tuesday, 10 p.m.) 21st Evac Hospital, Pusan. Excerpts of Virginia Taylor's letter to her parents:

Returned yesterday from a trip to Wonju on the East Coast. Slept all day yesterday and last night, so am raring to go again today. The news this a.m. has the Marines on <u>Bunker Hill</u> fighting furiously again, so I guess we'll be heading North again real soon. It has been rainy now for 3 weeks and the weather cool.

My Rest & Recuperation (R&R) has finally come around and will be getting 7 days leave to Japan toward the last of the month. I expected to go last May or June, but the personnel couldn't be spared at that time. I will get all my Christmas shopping done and send everyone a nice gift from Japan.

Most of my crew is leaving Korea in December or January. We have all worked for 9 months together. <u>I could possibly come home next month, but have asked to stay until the crew leaves.</u> As much as I'd like to come home, I feel that my time, while in the Army, will be more useful here, where one really feels he is needed and useful. <u>Three or four months out of a lifetime isn't too much to give to this mess.</u>

During 1952, nagging problems emerged as the draft and rotation interacted. Command experience was at a premium as veterans departed. Nurses were too few, Medical Service Corps officers were abundant but short on experience, and trained enlisted people were difficult to come by.[51]

After Virginia Taylor extended her rotation, <u>she had worked a total of 18 months on the hospital trains</u>. Combined with her arrival to Okinawa in June 1950, she had spent <u>over two-and a-half</u> years in the Far East—all related to the Korean War.

6138 AU Hospital Train
APO 301

13 August 1952

SUBJECT: Letter of Commendation

TO: Commanding Officer
421 Medical Collecting Company
APO 301

1. I wish to express my appreciation and gratitude for the service rendered by the six medical corpsman from your organization, listed below, who have been assigned to Hospital Train Number 105.

Hawley, Selby L.	Cpl US	Assist Crewchief
Costa, Roy W.	Cpl US	Corpsman
Jackson, Charles C.	Cpl US	Corpsman
Tate, Newell H.	Pfc US	Corpsman
Mosher, Louis O.	Pfc US	Corpsman
McCray, Willie	Pfc US	Corpsman

2. The Commanding Officer or Train Commander renders the ratings and efficiency reports on the men, but it is the nurse who knows best the qualities and capacities of each man.

3. It is seldom that one finds a group of men who worked with as much team work and harmony as the crew of train number 105.

4. Five of these men had charge of a hospital coach, each carrying 36 sick and wounded patients, one has worked as assistant crewchief for the past 8 months.

5. These men are leaders and each played a key part on our Hospital Train. I do not hesitate when I say that they are the finest group of corpsman that I have ever worked with. Although I can do nothing about the "Whys" and "Wherefores" of the Army, it is with great reluctance that I give them back to you. Their loss will leave a great vacancy.

VIRGINIA E. TAYLOR/ 1st Lt
Nurse in Charge, Hosp. Train #105

1st Lt. Virginia Taylor's COMMENDATION for her corpsmen

9 Sept 1952
Tuesday
10 pm

Dearest Folks,

Returned yesterday from a trip to Wonju on the East coast. Slept all day yesterday & last night so am raring to go again today. The news this a.m. has the Marines on Bunker Hill fighting furiously again so I guess we'll be heading North again real soon. It has been raining now for 3 weeks and the weather cool.

My Rest & Recuperation (R & R) has finally come around and will be getting 7 days leave to Japan toward the last of this month. I expected to go last May or June but the personnel couldn't be spared at that time. I will get all my Christmas shopping done & send everyone a nice gift from Japan.

Most of my crew are leaving Korea in December & January. We have all worked for 9 months together and hope to all go home together. I possibly could come home next month but have asked to to stay until the crew leaves. As much as I'd like to come home, I feel that my time, while in the Army, will be more useful here, where one really feels he is needed and useful. 3 or 4 extra months out of a lifetime isn't too much to give to this mess.

That Income tax I knew I was going to have to pay as they forgot to take it out for one month when I first came to Korea. I'm glad the foundation for the house is going up. I'll be able to help with a lot when I get home.

Ruth sure is getting to be quite a lady. Does she have everything she needs for school?

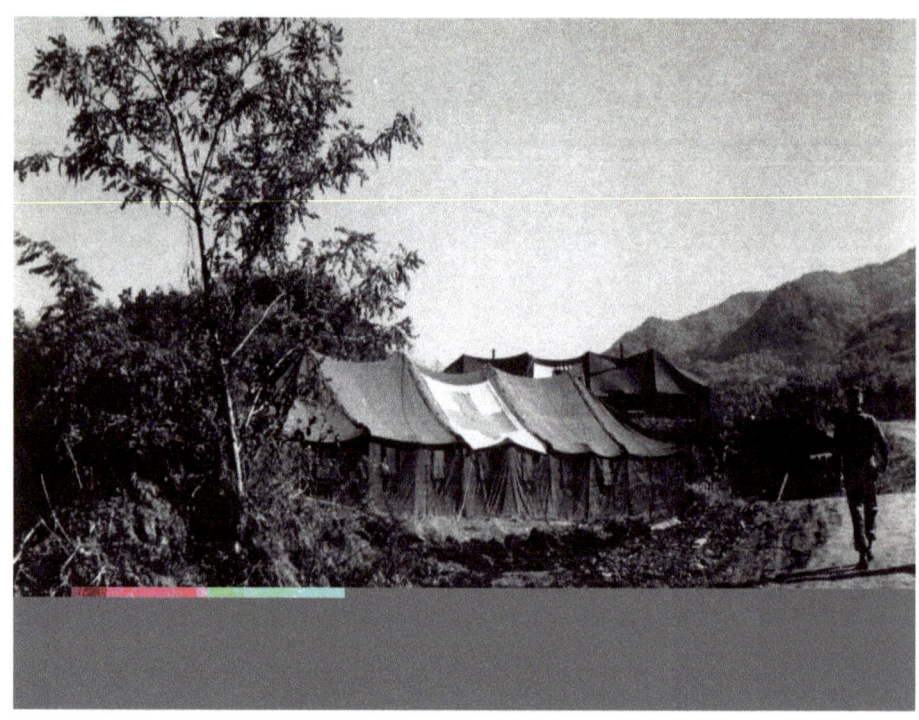

Sintanni 2nd Div Collecting Station
(8,000 yards from the enemy lines)

(Photo courtesy of Virginia Taylor collection)

October 22, 1952 (Wednesday, 8 p.m.), Pusan. Excerpts of Virginia Taylor's letter to her parents: (Note: Sonny was Virginia's brother)

Returned from the north yesterday afternoon—had a letter from you and Sonny. Figured I'd sit down and be a answering while the wind's a howling outside and our oil heater is giving off with the warmth.

The fighting the past 3 weeks has really been rough. Whole companies have been wiped out on <u>White Horse.</u> The ROKs Korean Army have taken the heaviest fighting. A Hospital Train loads at Sintanni every 24 hours.

Sintanni was within 8,000 yards of the frontlines and approximately 30 miles above the 38th Parallel in North Korea.

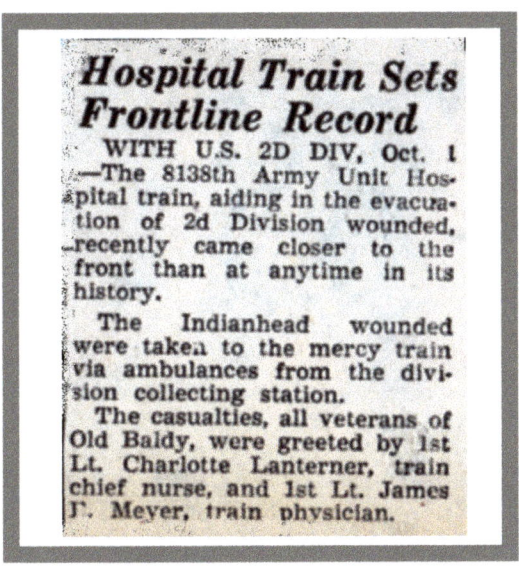

Courtesy of Virginia Taylor collection)[52]

The time for us all goes fast when we are busy. I guess it'll be Christmas before we know it. Tomorrow Evelyn and I teach English class to two Korean girls. One is studying to be a doctor. Dr. Kim age 20 and the other, her sister. They want to both help their people.

22 October 1952
Wednesday
8 pm

Dearest Folks,

Returned from the north yesterday afternoon - had a letter from you & Sonny. Figured I'd get set down and be a answering while the winds a howling outside and our oil heater is giving off with the warmth.

The fighting the past 3 weeks has really been rough. Whole company have been wiped out on "White Horse." The ROK's Korean Army have taken the heaviest fighting. A Hospital Train load at Sintanni every 24 hours.

The Time forges all goes fast when you are busy I guess it'll be Christmas before we know it.

I am going to get all my summer uniforms boxed up & send them home. Also all the other stuff I got hanging around so's when I get my orders I can travel light.

It is now 10:20. We just came back from the movie "The Winning Team" with Doris Day. For once the machine didn't break down or the power fail.

Tomorrow Evelyn & I teach English class to two Korean girls. One is studying to be a doctor - Dr Kim - age 20 & the other her sister - They want to both

December 1, 1952. Excerpts of Virginia Taylor's letter to her sister (Rosie): (Note: Train Nurse: Betty Potocik is mentioned in this letter.)

I am glad you got to talk with Betty. She is sure a No. 1 Gal. Received a letter from her today also. She said you sounded just like me, and if she hadn't had such short time, would have visited with you. She is going to be stationed at West Point. Her first choice was Fort Jay on Governors Island. She had chosen West Point for her second preference.

I'm choosing Letterman as 1st, 2nd, and 3rd choice. If they don't assign me there, I will be most unhappy. I could go home on days off and could be a big help to the Folks. I have one more year left to serve in the A.N.C., then I'm going to get out and go to school I think.

The fighting here in Korea has quieted, and a great lull has settled over the Front. Everyone is waiting for General Eisenhower's arrival. All units have specially prepared banners, signs, flags, parades, etc. The general feeling about IKE over here is that a change certainly couldn't hurt the present stalemate. Maybe he will have a solution.

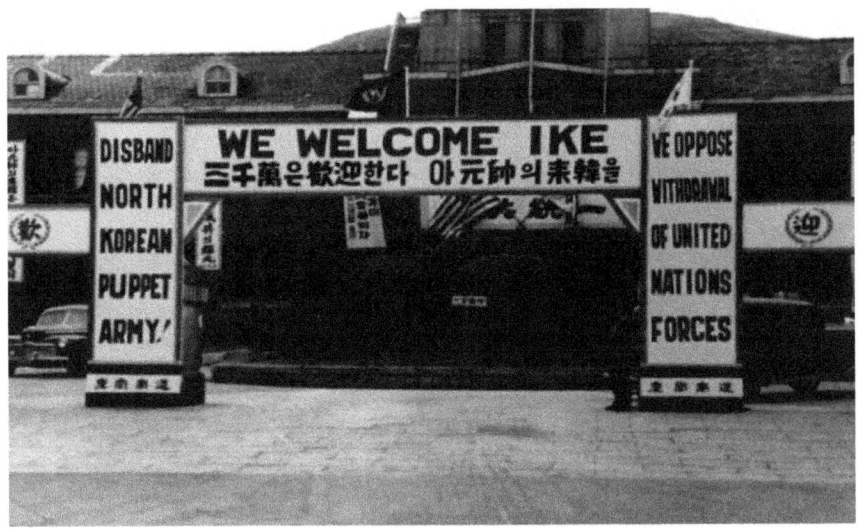

(Photo courtesy Virginia Taylor collection)

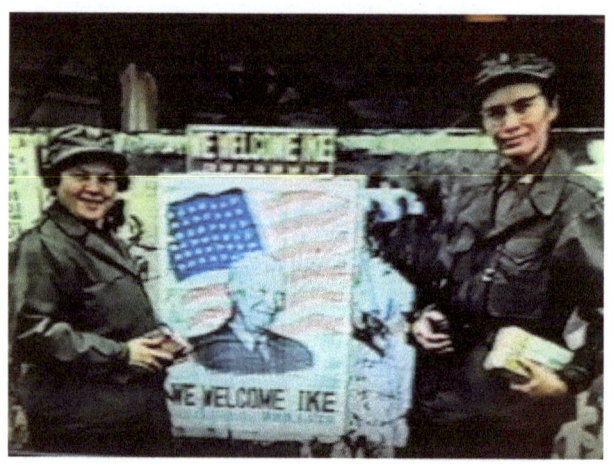

Lts Corrine Bryant and Virginia Taylor in front of WELCOME "IKE" sign

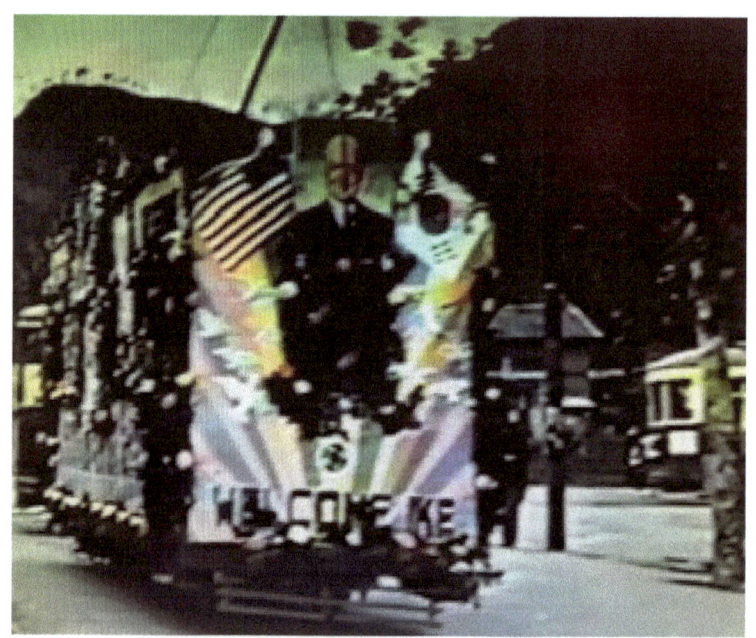

U.N. Day: Decorated Streetcar
(Photos courtesy of Virginia Taylor collection)

*During the month of October occurred the heaviest, bitterest fighting of the Korean War. Of the Hospital trains, 105 carried the highest number of casualties—**3,090 in one month**. On one trip we had them sitting in sinks, laying on stoves, piled up in cupboards, shower room floors—3 to 4 to a bed and every place except hanging from the ceiling. Our capacity is 216. That day we loaded with 469.*

At present, we go as far north as Sintanni—4 miles from Chorwon and no man's land. An occasional round of artillery falls near, but so far none of the hospital trains have been hit. Lt. Potociks train, 103 was attacked in October by enemy soldiers dressed as South Korean guards. They shot up the engine and engineer, but American troops got there before they could get inside the train.

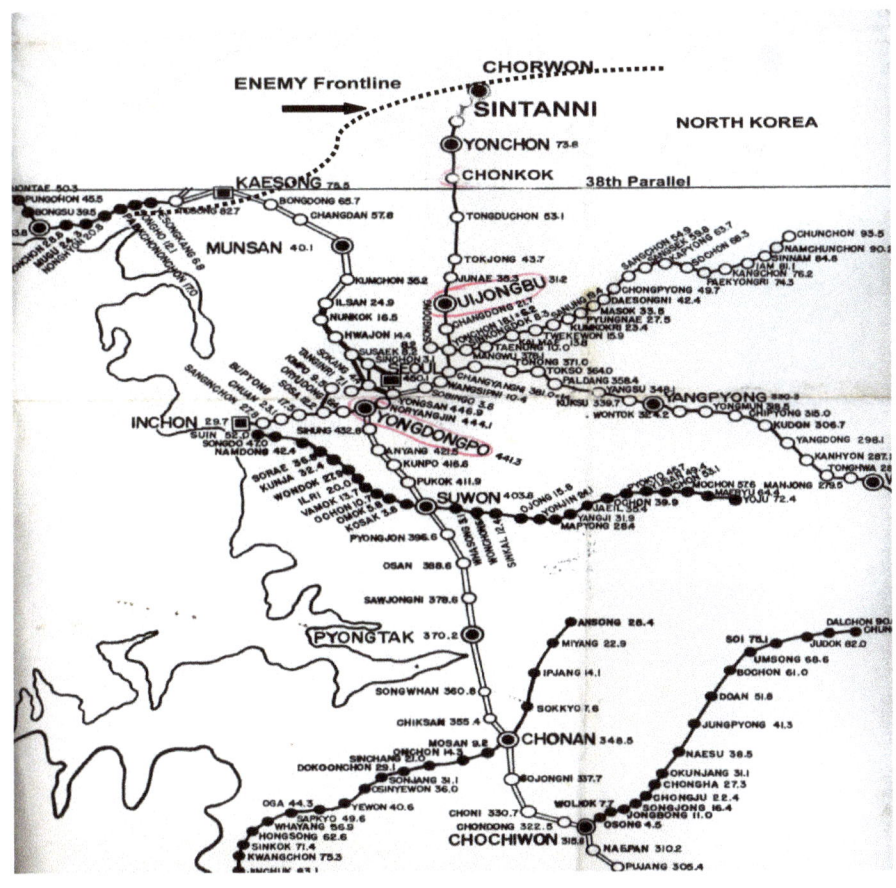

(RR Map—courtesy of Virginia Taylor collection)

You asked if any newsreels had been taken of anything I was near. An Army photographer took newsreels of the <u>train wreck where 200 school kids were injured and 20 killed. Hospital Train 105 was just a mile away from the tragedy and we were called over. The crew and I and an Army doctor cut off 3 legs and 2 arms that day.</u> I could hear cameras grinding and clicking but had no time to see what was going on. We got a special letter from the Commanding Officer for giving the medical assistance that we did. That's been 2 or 3 months ago, but maybe they might show the newsreels somewhere.

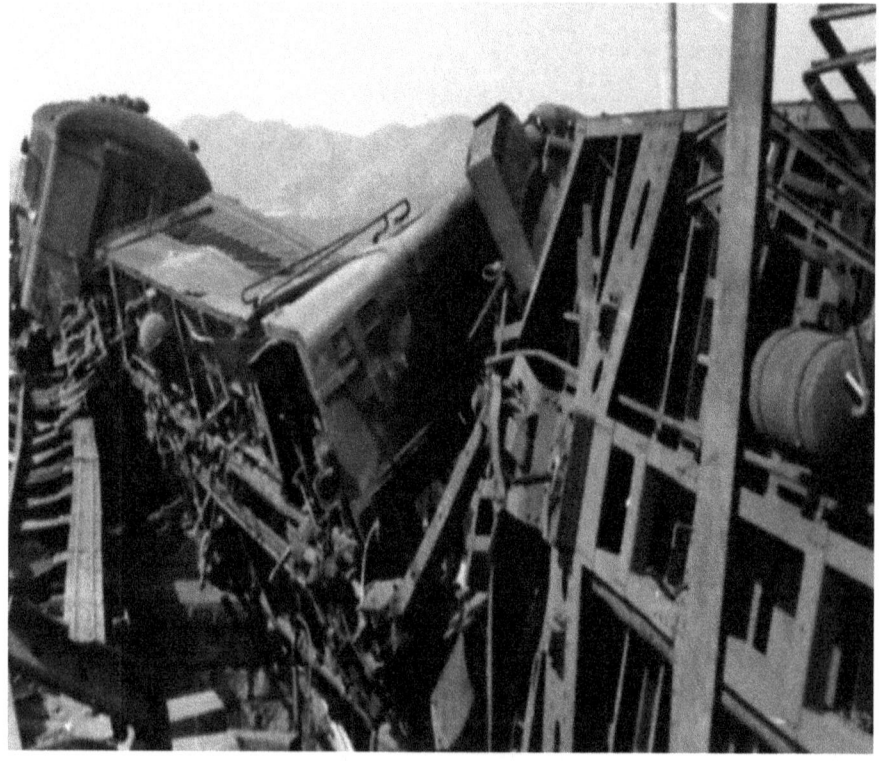

(Photo courtesy Virginia Taylor collection)

TWISTED CARS CLOG BRIDGE
200 INJURED

YONGDONPO, September 17, 1952 (Pacific S&S)—A railway bridge closed by this sprawling industrial suburb of Seoul was an appalling scene this morning after the tender of a train carrying hundreds of Korean school children blew up.

Even veterans of battle who hurried to the area said they had never seen a sight more gruesome. The three coaches of the train lay twisted across the length of the bridge under a bright September sun. But there was blood—and possibly more bodies—in the muddy water below.

AT LEAST 11 of the youngsters were believed killed in the wreck. No one could say how many kids were on the train but one soldier on the scene said, "there must have been five or six hundred." An estimated 200 were hurt.

BY EARLY afternoon, the last tot believed to be alive under the crumpled mass of metal had been removed. But it was an operation that shocked and stabbed everyone who was close enough to hear the little girl's heart-rendering screams as an Army medical officer, working under the worst possible conditions for emergency surgery cut her loose from the wreckage with a hook saw.

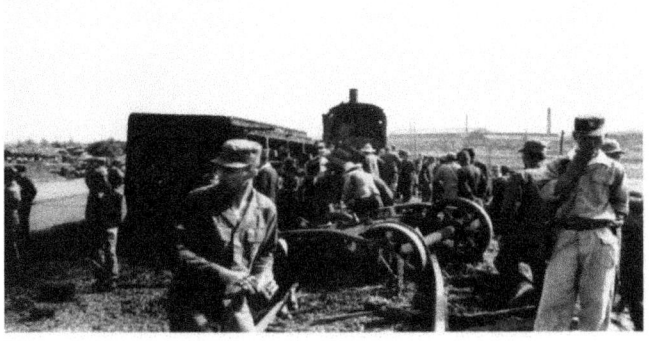

(Photo courtesy Virginia Taylor collection)

TWISTED CARS CLOG BRIDGE
(Continued)

Her shrill wails and moans, "mother, mother," went on for what seemed an interminable time for the medics, streaming with sweat and splattered with blood, who finally extricated her from the crushing weight of the coach. Her right arm had been pinned under at the shoulder. <u>Now she only had one shoulder.</u>

FROM THE CENTRAL car of the wrecked train, a small pair of legs dangled. "It's a little boy," said one officer on the scene. "We'll get him out later—we know he's dead."

One of the witness to the crackup—PTE John Clarke of Berkshire, England, said the ripped coaches poured hundreds of children into the shallow water below the bridge.

"They came swarming up the banks, they were screaming and crying and falling down. They were all cut up and bloody and they didn't know what had happened," said Clarke. "It was the most horrible thing I have ever seen, you could hear the awful moans and shrieks from under the cars where the other kids were trapped."

Army medics from the 121st Evacuation Hospital and the 45th Division were knocking themselves out to relieve suffering from 8 a.m. on into the afternoon when the last living child was cut loose from the wreckage.

Captain Alfred M. Bennett of Chicago, a Thunderbird medical officer, said, "One or two" of the kids died enroute to the hospital after being taken from the train.

Excerpt from the letter below:

As the only nurse present, you did splendid work during the disaster. Without your tireless efforts, your cool cooperation and assistance to the medical officers, the casualties may have been higher.

HEADQUARTERS
Hospital Train, 8138th Army Unit
APO 301

22 September 1952

SUBJECT: Letter of Appreciation

TO: 1st Lt Virginia M. Taylor
N 804 301

1. Following the tragic disaster of the Korean school train at Oryu-Dong near Yong Dong Po on 17 September 1952 during which twenty (20) school children lost their lives and in excess of two hundred (200) were injured, I wish to express to you my particular commendation and gratitude.

2. As the only nurse present, you did splendid work during the disaster. Without your tireless efforts, your cool cooperation and assistance to the medical officers, the casualties may have been higher.

3. Your efforts reflected great credit not only upon yourself, but also upon the Army Nurse Corps and the 8138th AU, Hospital Train.

GERHARD J. NEWERIA
Captain MC
Commanding

Twisted Cars Clog Bridge; 200 Injured

By M/Sgt. Bill FitzGerald

YONGDONGPO, Sept. 17 (Pac. S&S)—A railway bridge close by this sprawling industrial suburb of Seoul was an appalling scene this morning after the tender of a train carrying hundreds of Korean school children blew up.

Even veterans of battle who hurried to the area said they had never seen a sight more gruesome. The three coaches of the train lay twisted across the length of the bridge under a bright September sun. But there was blood—and possibly more bodies—in the muddy water below.

AT LEAST 11 of the youngsters were believed killed in the wreck. No one could say how many kids were on the train, but one soldier on the scene said "there must have been five or six hundred." An estimated 200 were hurt.

BY EARLY afternoon the last tot believed to be alive under the crumpled mass of metal had been removed. But it was an operation that shocked and stabbed everyone who was close enough to hear the little girl's heart-rendering screams as an Army medical officer, working under the worst possible conditions for emergency surgery, cut her loose from the wreckage with a hook saw.

Her shrill wails and moans, "mother, mother," went on for what seemed an interminable time for medics, streaming with sweat and splattered with blood, who finally extricated her from the crushing weight of the coach. Her right arm had been pinned under at the shoulder. Now she had only a shoulder.

FROM THE CENTRAL car of the wrecked train, a small pair of legs dangled. "It's a little boy," said one officer on the scene. "We'll get him out later —we know he's dead."

One witness to the crackup— Pte. John Clarke of Berkshire, England, said the ripped coaches poured hundreds of children into the shallow water below the bridge.

"They came swarming up the banks, they were screaming and crying and falling down. They were all cut up and bloody and they didn't know what had happened," said Clarke. "It was the most horrible thing I have ever seen, you could hear the awful moans and shrieks from under the cars where the other kids were trapped."

Army medics from the 121st Evacuation Hospital and the

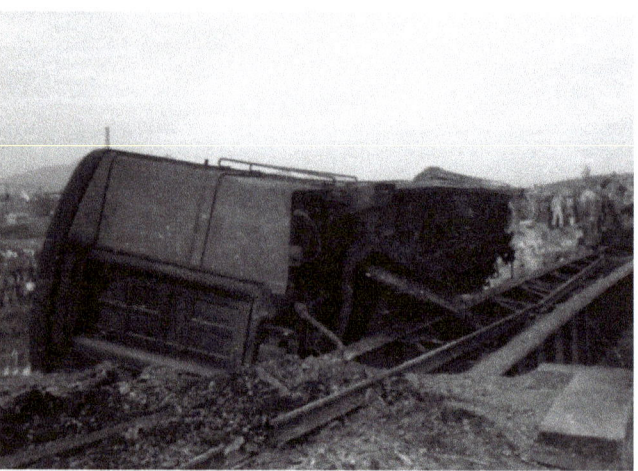

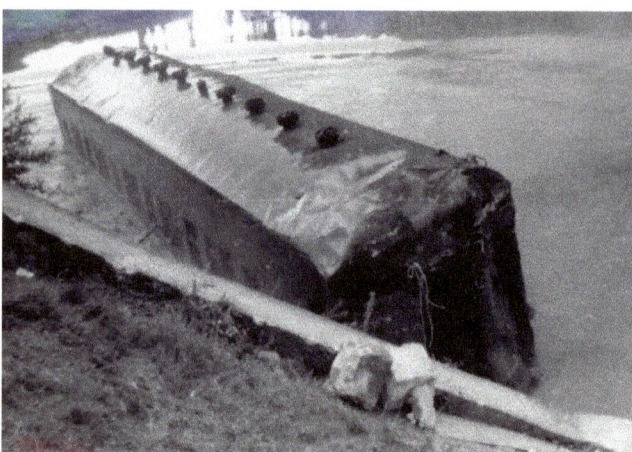

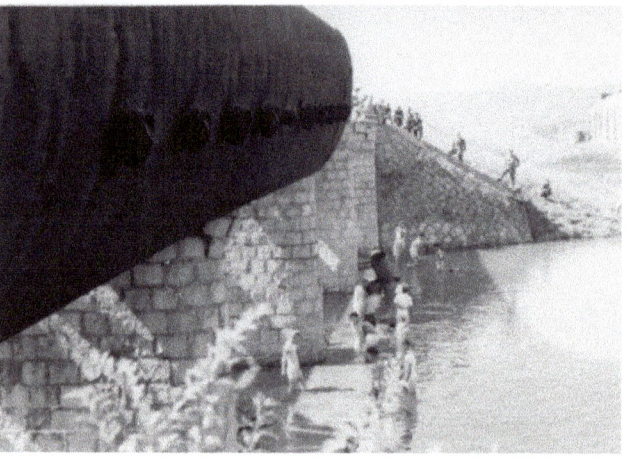

(Photos courtesy of Virginia Taylor collection)

A Postcard from Virginia's brother (2005)

Rose clarified about Ginger's Korea war record: That the worst hospital train trip was in 1952 <u>when 50 or more of the U.S. wounded out of 200 total died before the train reached Pusan</u>. (Hospital ships there.)

On the trip when the enemy blew up the trestle, 50 Korean (South) were killed when their flat car fell into the river.

One car of schoolchildren was saved when the engine stopped just in time. Another car of 50 children fell with 20 killed.

Virginia, being the strongest of the nurses, carried four kids out separately. The medics (and Virginia) had to carry the injured children. Then, the medics and Virginia agreed to "adopt" one child each, and they all had $20 per month taken out of their pay.

Virginia continued to write to her eight-year-old "adopted" Korean child for five more years. When her Army pay stopped after her Masters from Stanford University (1956), she invited the girl to the U.S.

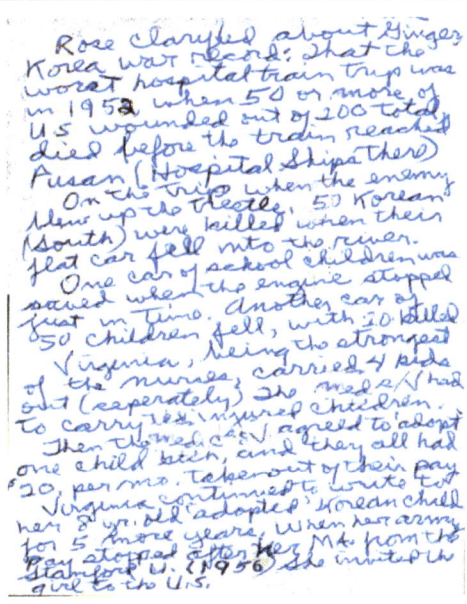

It is going to be a cold winter looks like. Snow has already fallen up north and old Papasans rice fields are covered over with ice and frost.

Thousands of little children are still without homes or food or clothes and thousand will die this winter. Life is so cheap here. No one cares except the Americans and the need is so great that what help we give seems to just scratch the surface.

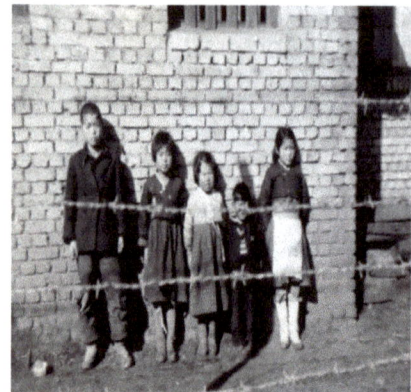 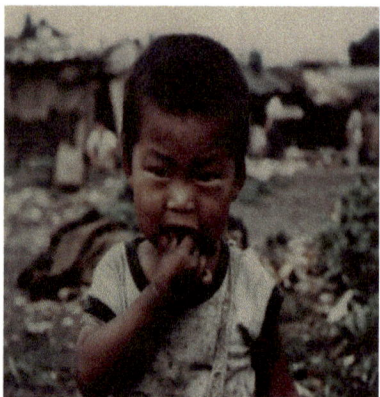

(Photos courtesy of Virginia Taylor collection)

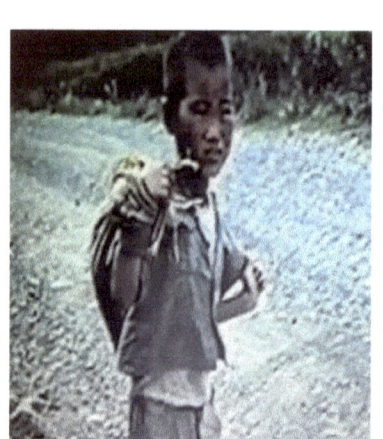 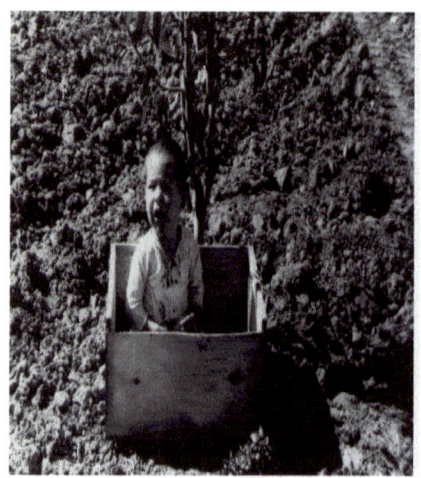

This experience has been good—as I shall NEVER again grumble or complain. The misery, heartache, and suffering of this tragic land will always be with me.

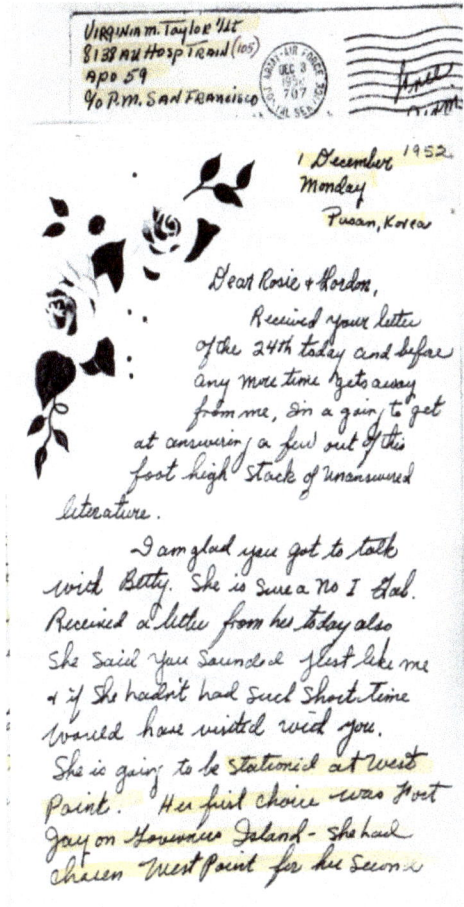

1 December 1952
Monday
Pusan, Korea

Dear Rosie & Gordon,

Received your letter of the 24th today and before any more time gets away from me, I'm going to get at answering a few out of this foot high stack of unanswered literature.

I am glad you got to talk with Betty. She is sure a No 1 Gal. Received a letter from her today also. She said you sounded just like me & if she hadn't had such short time would have visited with you. She is going to be stationed at West Point. Her first choice was Fort Jay on Governors Island—she had chosen West Point for her second preference. I am choosing Letterman as 1st, 2nd & 3rd. If they don't assign me there I will be most unhappy. I could go home on days off & could be of a big help to the folks. I have one more year left to serve in the A.N.C. Then I'm going to get out & go to school I think.

The fighting here in Korea has quieted and a great lull has settled over the front. Everyone is waiting for Gen'l Eisenhower's arrival. All units have specially prepared banners, signs, flags, parades etc. The general feeling about Ike over here is that a change certainly can't hurt the present stalemate here. Maybe he will have a solution.

II

During the month of October occurred the heaviest, bitterest fighting of the Korean War. Of the Hospital Trains — 105 carried the higest no of casualties — 3090 in one month. On one trip we had them sitting in sinks, laying on stoves, piled up in cupboards, shower rooms, floors — 3 & 4 to a bed and everyplace except hanging from the celing. Our capacity is 216, that day we loaded with 469. Now we barely have enough for one coach — (36 patients) for which we are all thankful.

At present we go as far north as Sintanni — 4 miles from chorwon and no mans land. An occasional round of artillary falls near but so far none of the Hospital trains have been hit. Lt Potocki's Train, 103, was attacked one night in October by enemy soldiers dressed as South Korean Guards. They shot up the engine & engineer but American troops got there before they could get inside the train.

You asked if any news reels had been taken of anything I was near. An Army photographer took Newsreels of the Train wreck where 200 School kids were injured & 20 killed. Hosp Train 105, my train, was just a mile away from the tragedy and we were called over. The crew & I & an army Dr cut off 3 legs & 2 arms that day. I could hear cameras

III

grinding & clicking but had no time to see what was going on. We all got a special letter from the commander office for giving the medical assistance that we did. That's been 2 or 3 months ago but maybe they might show the newsreels somewhere.

It is going to be a cold winter looks like. Snow has already fallen up North and old papa san's Rice fields are covered over with ice & frost.

Thousands of little children are still without homes or food or clothes & thousands will die this winter. Life is so cheap here no one cares except the Americans and the need is so great that what help we give seems to just scratch the surface. This experience has been good - as I shall never again grumble or complain. The misery, heartache and suffering of this tragic land will always be with me.

Well enough of this carrying on — you are probably getting tired of trying to decipher my chicken tracks so will close for now. Write soon & give my love to all.

P.S. The scarf was bought in Korea — a shop in Seoul. I sent some dolls & a musical pipe of what ever else is in there to this mob will post week for for you & kids

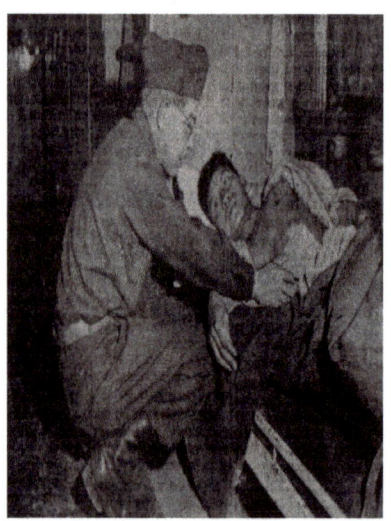

8138 AU HOSPITAL TRAIN COMMANDER
Captain (Doctor) Gerhard Newerla

HEADQUARTERS
Hospital Train, 8138th Army Unit
APO 301

10 November 1952

SUBJECT: Letter of Commendation

FROM: Commanding Officer
8138th Army Unit Hospital Train
APO 301

TO: All Members of my Command.

Upon entering the hospital for possible evacuation because of ill health, I wish to take this opportunity to thank all members of my command, including those from the 217th Medical Collecting Co and the 765th Railway Shop Battalion, for the loyal support you have given me.

No organization can be better than the officers and men who comprise it. I have always been proud of you and considered our Hospital Train Unit the finest in Korea. Your loyalty, devotion to duty and efficiency, often associated with great difficulties and long hours, has been exceptional. Without your help we could not have performed our mission of mercy as well as we did. You all deserve and should be proud of the Meritorious Unit Citation which you have earned.

Keep up this good work in the future, especially when the going should become harder.

I salute and commend you.

GERHARD J. NEWERLA
Captain   MC
Commanding

LETTER OF COMMENDATION
From Captain Gerhard Newerla
(Courtesy of Virginia Taylor collection)

CHONKOK 618TH CLEARING STATION, NORTH KOREA
10 miles above the 38th parallel

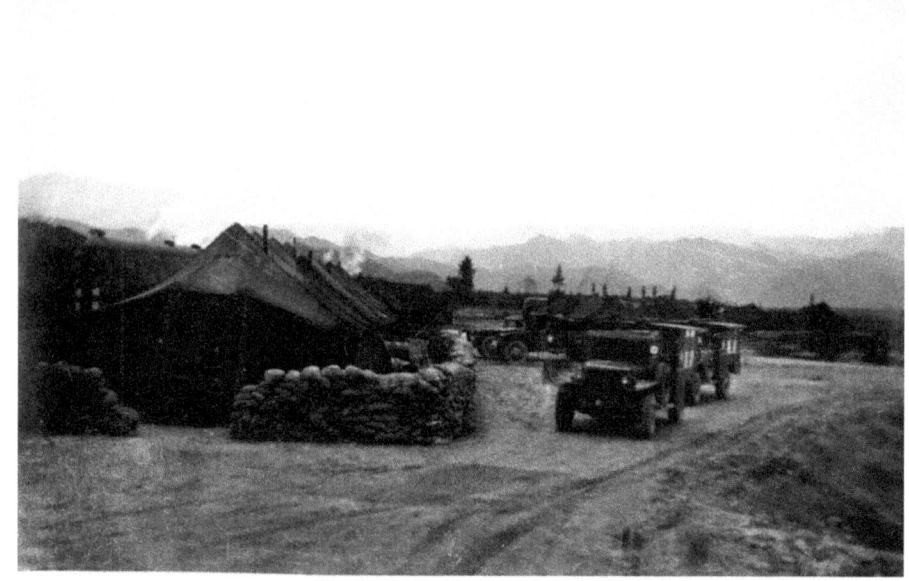

DECEMBER 25, 1952. Cold gray CHRISTMAS DAY. Ambulances from the 8055 MASH. Note the steam coming from TRAIN 105 (left).
(Photo courtesy of Virginia Taylor collection)

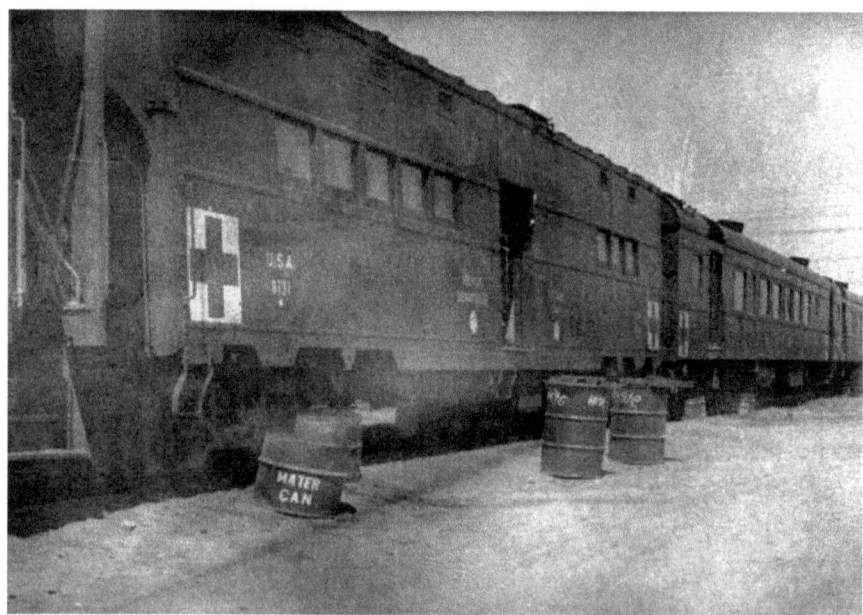

TRAIN 106 (Kitchen Car) at a water point. (The 712th Railway Operating Battalion (TROB) maintained water cans along the rail route).
(Photo courtesy of Don Verstraete collection)

A WOUNDED MAN COMES BACK
AS THE SOLDIER SEES IT

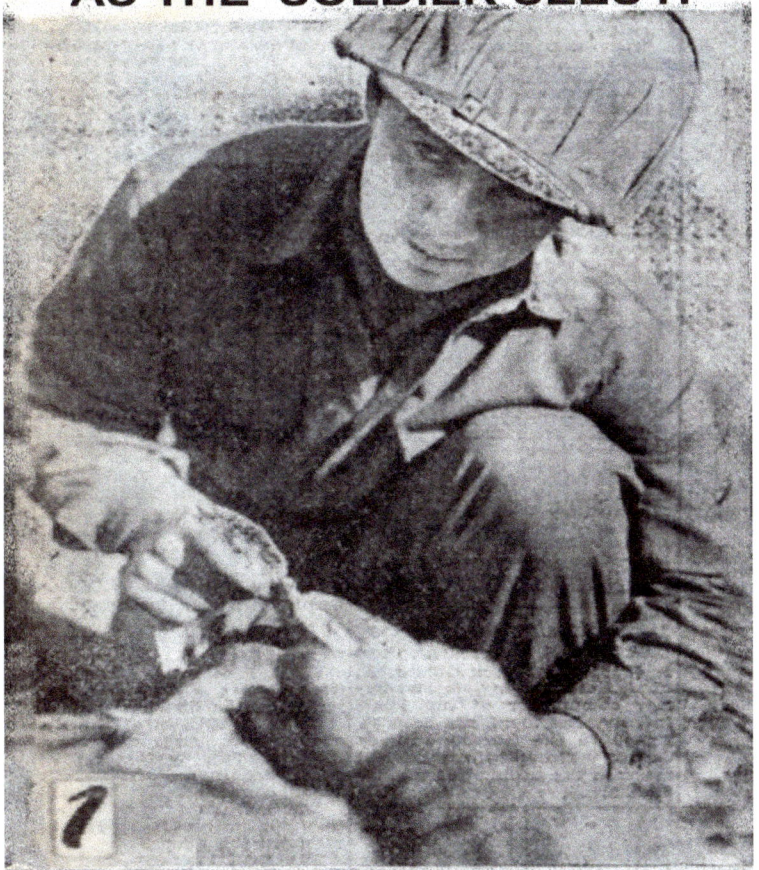

1. FRONTLINE AIDMAN PFC Ronald Gilbert Munkelwitz, 2d Infantry Division, dresses my "wound" at an outpost on the central front.

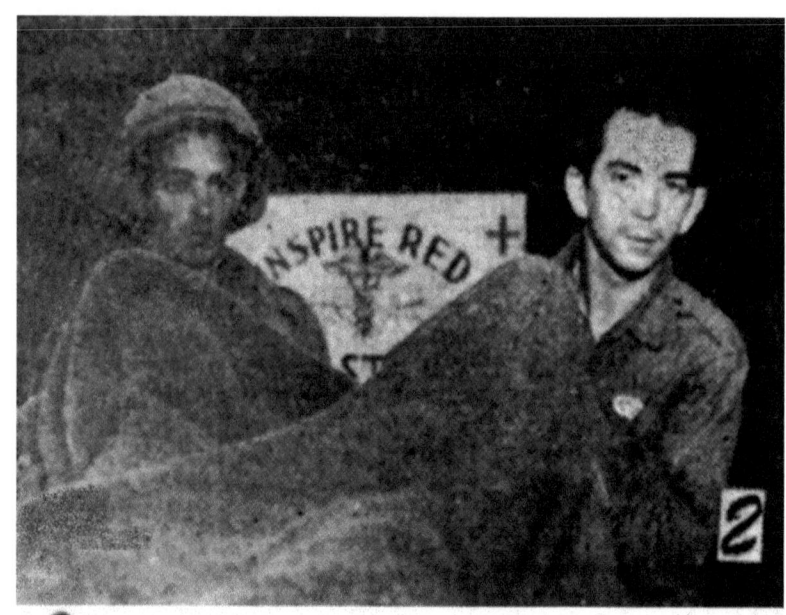

2. I AM UNLOADED from a litter jeep after a mile and a half trip over the ridge from the outpost where I first received emergency aid. Holding the bottom of my litter are jeep driver PFC George H. Kent (left), Providence, R.I., and medic Sgt. John G. Patterson.

3. LIFE SAVING PLASMA begins flowing into my veins at the battalion aid station. The "doctor," 1st Lt. William E. Brock, starts the flow of the plasma after having checked my "wound." Medical corpsman Sergeant Patterson is assisting with the precious fluid.

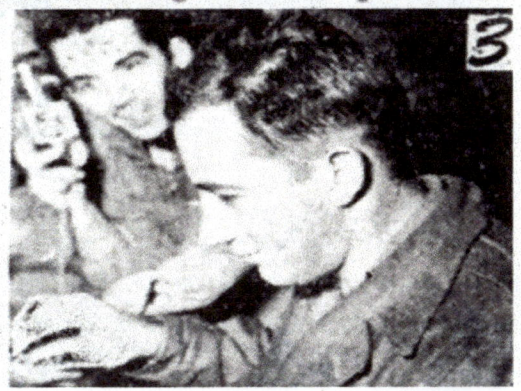

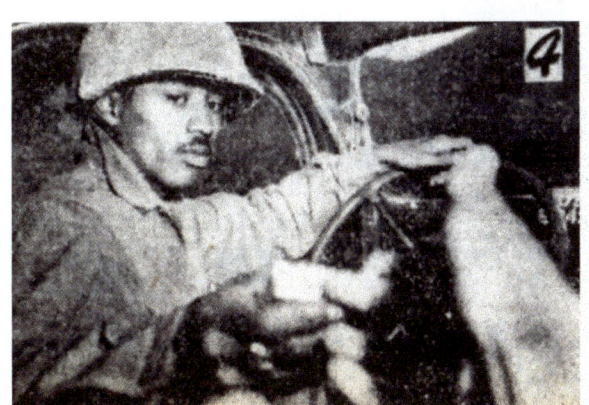

4. "THANKS, PAL," is what I mumble to ambulance driver PFC William Washington as he gives me a cigaret as we start the ambulance trip back to a 2d Infantry Division medical clearing station. Washington makes the trip rapidly, but cautiously for the sake of the wounded men.

5. MORPHINE, administered at division clearing station, begins to take effect on me and the division surgeon goes in and out of focus as he checks my heart and begins to administer whole blood.

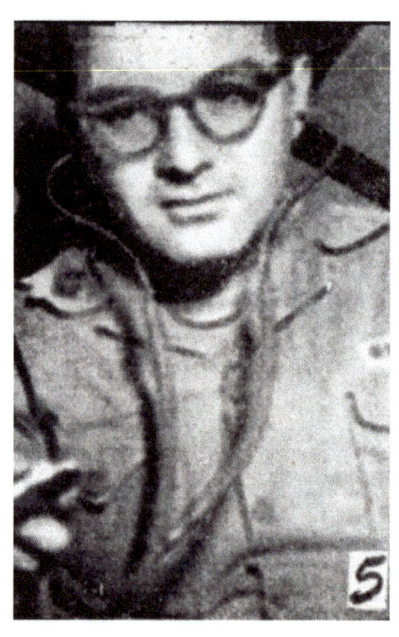

6. PLACED IN A HELICOPTER "POD" I look up and see "chopper" pilot, 1st Lt. Thurman Lawrence of the 3d Air Rescue Squadron. The quick, smooth air evacuation will get me back to a mobile Army surgical hospital for more treatment.

7 THE MASK COMES DOWN and soon I am in a painless sleep as the MASH surgeons begin to repair the damage. After final preparations the mask slipped over my face. Left to right are Capt. Richard Kamil, surgeon; Lt. Helen Black, anaesthetist, Capt. Ruth Kegler, operating room nurse, and PFC George Scott, operating room technician.

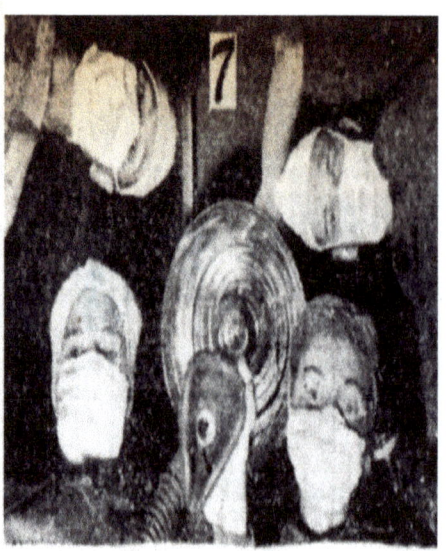

8. **LOVELY SIGHT** to greet a guy as he comes out of the ether in post operation section is nurse, 1st Lt. Elden F. Gubics. Her smile and cheerful manner tells me everything is "just lovely." I'm still not feeling too good, but she makes everything seem a little better.

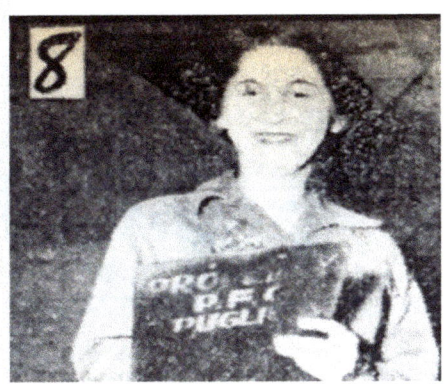

9. **ABOARD A HOSPITAL TRAIN**, bound for the 121st evac hospital, I get the best of care with constant attention from doctors and nurses. Here I look up as train physician Lt. James E. Meyer, and nurse 1st Lt. Charlotte R. Lanternirer check my records during the four-hour train trip.

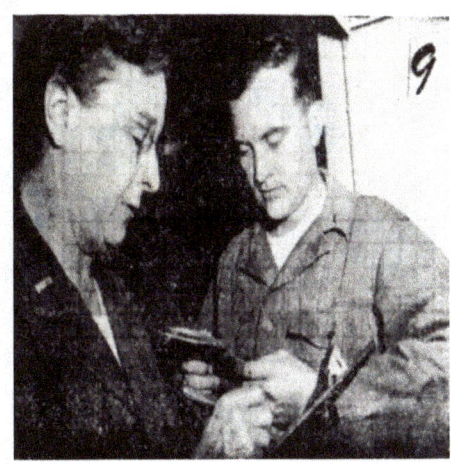

10. AFTER MY SECOND OPERATION in 36 hours, I wake up in the 121st evac to find I've been sleeping in a real bed and on honest to goodness, real, white sheets. I am watching Pvt. Robert H. Ellis, corpsman, and nurse 1st Lt. Doris H. Troy making some other patients comfortable.

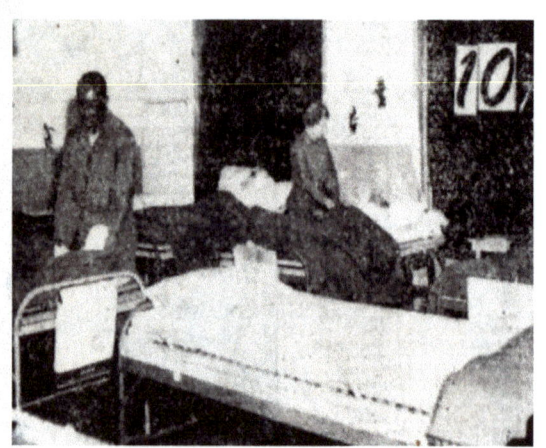

11. IN THE AIR I am aboard a C-54 winging its way back to a hospital in Japan. Three people help to make our flight more comfortable. They are flight nurse Victoria Malokas, medical technician Harry Karz, and A2/C William Grice, all of the 801st medical air evacuation service.

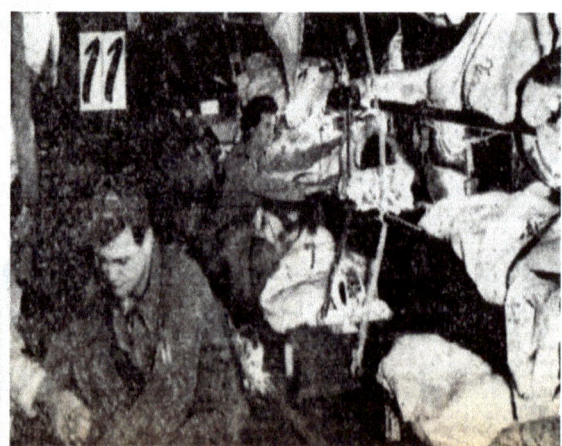

Virginia connected with her patients. Often, she would check on them days later as shown in the excerpt from her February 25, 1952 letter to her parents: *The frostbite (patient) you asked about was flown to Japan several days ago and was expected to lose only his toes.* In the pictures below, Virginia escorted a patient from the hospital train to the airfield to be transported by helicopter for immediate care.

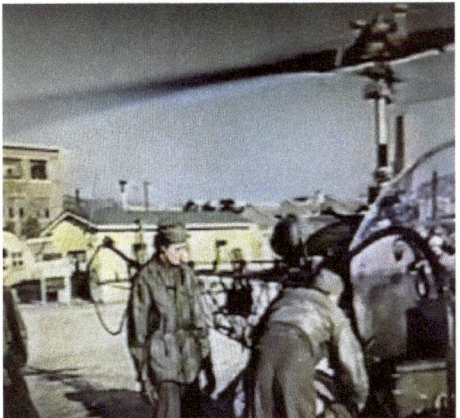
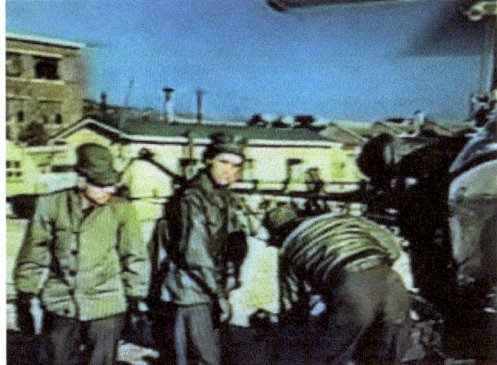

Nurse Virginia Taylor and Crew Chief Andy Anderson

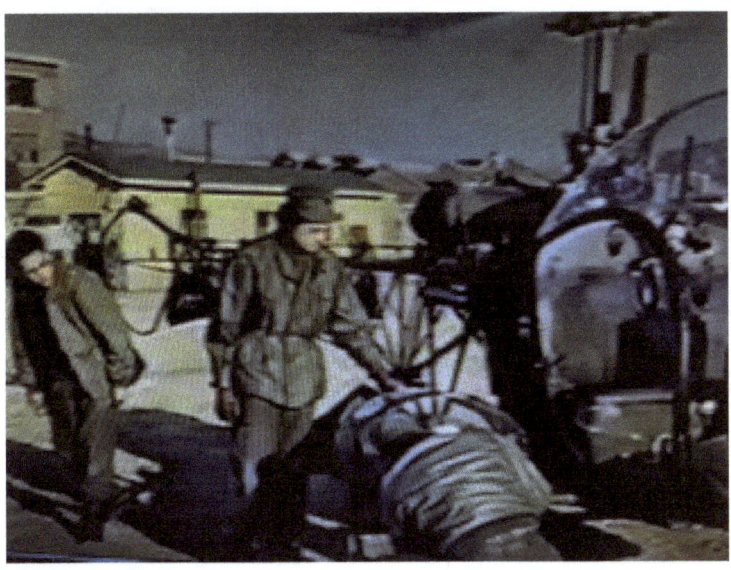

Note Virginia's hand on the carrier as if she is wishing the patient safe travels. (Photos courtesy of Virginia Taylor collection)

AIRFORCE RESCUE HELICOPTER

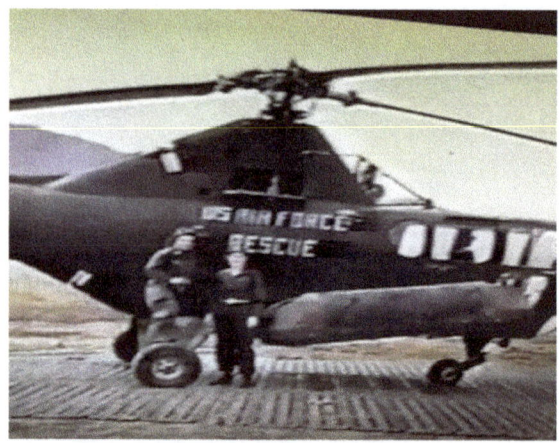

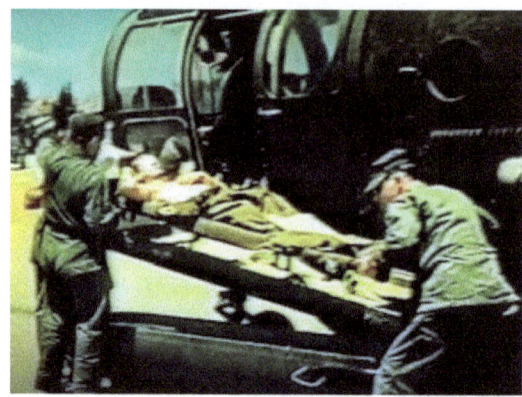

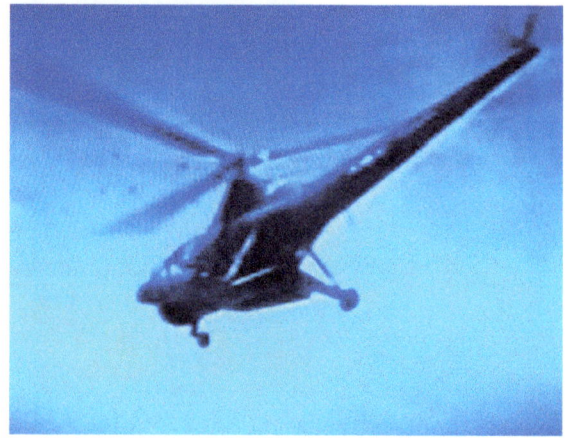

(Photos courtesy of Virginia Taylor collection)

THE AIRFIELDS

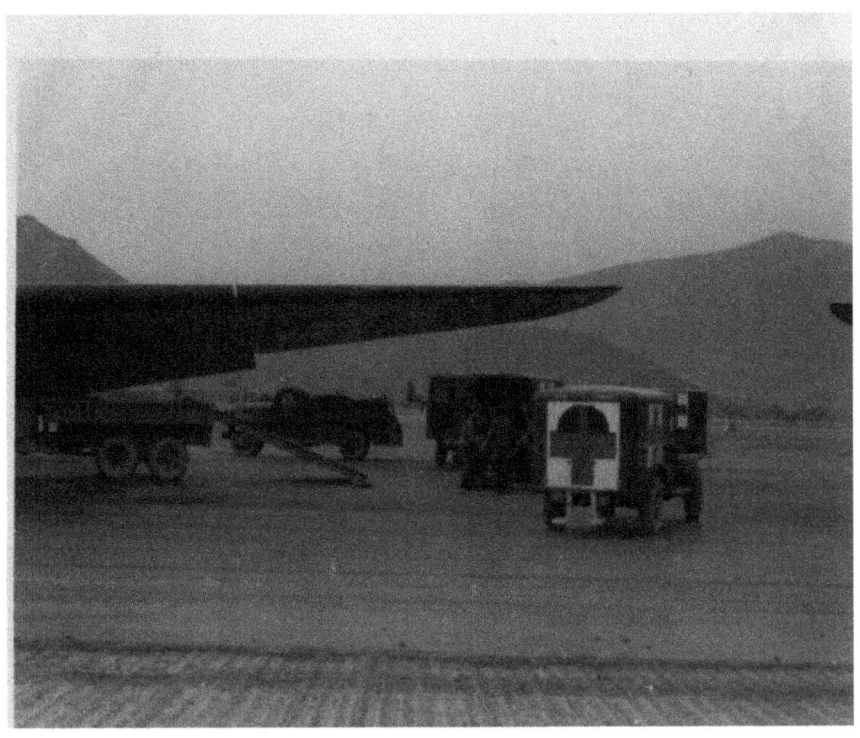

Medics loading patients onto planes

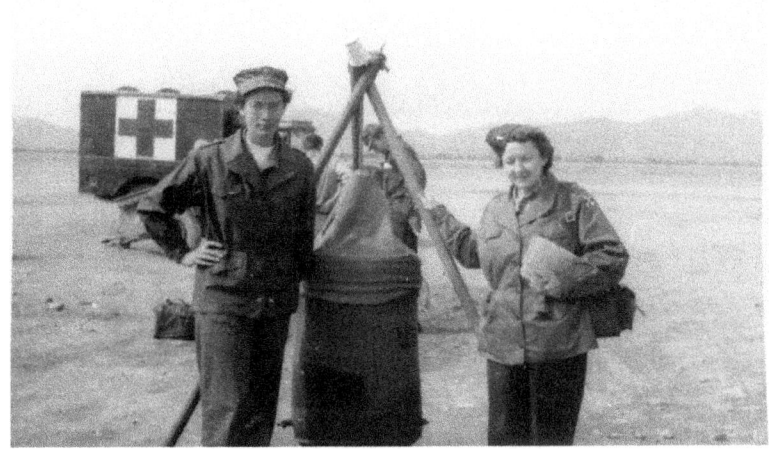

Lt. Virginia Taylor (Train 105) and Lt. Wade (Train 101)
K-1 Marine Airfield
(Photos courtesy of Virginia Taylor collection)

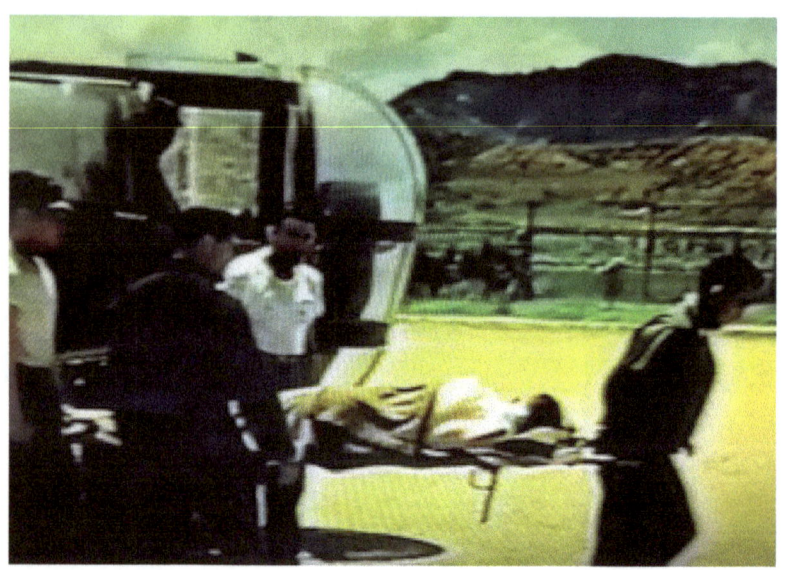

Transported from the front to 121st Evac Hospital in Yongdongpo

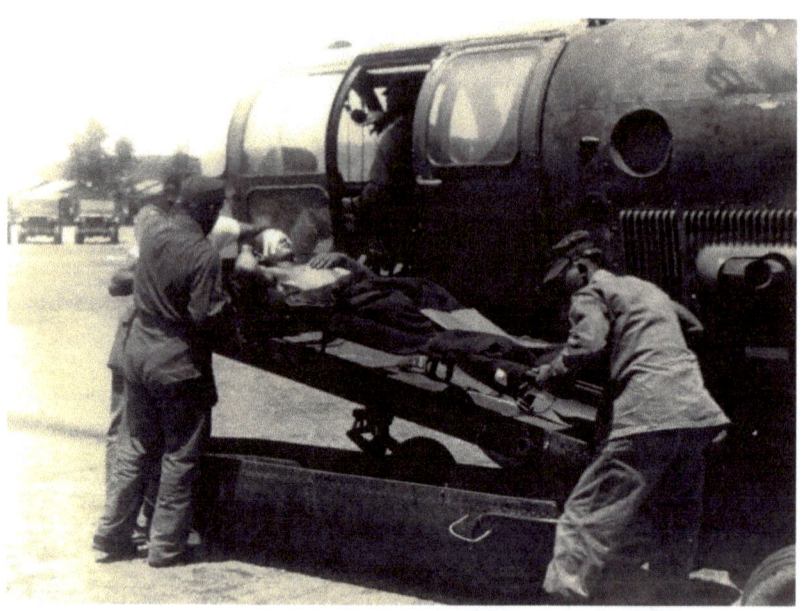

Taken from 121st EVAC Hospital (Yongdongpo) to a Navy hospital ship in Inchon Harbor for treatment by an eye specialist.

(Photos courtesy Virginia Taylor collection)

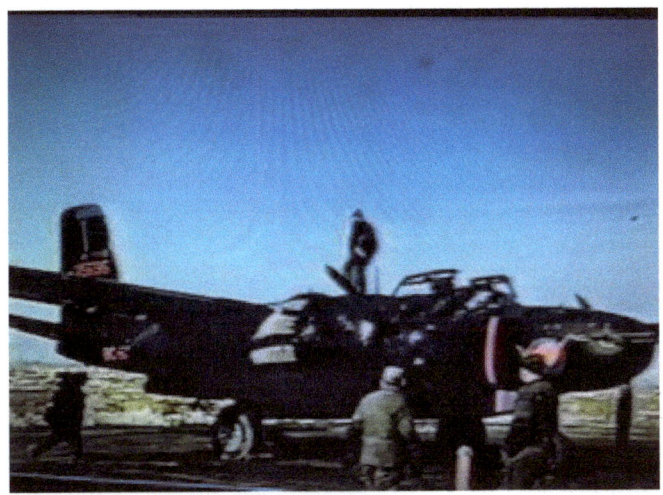

Fighter jet at airfield

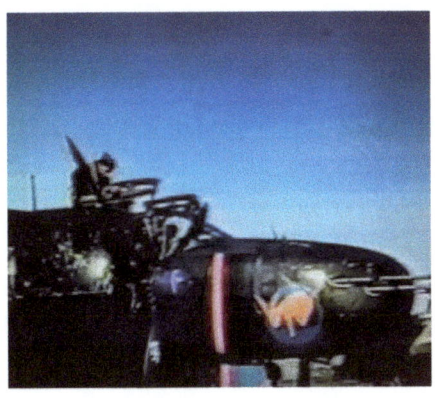

(Photos courtesy of Virginia Taylor collection)

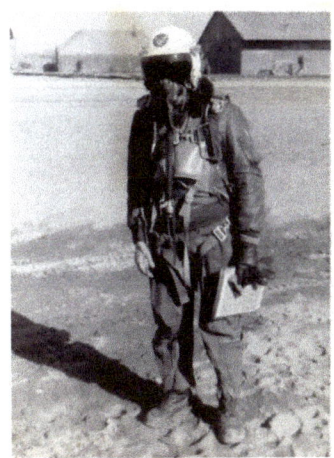

Sabre Jet pilot
(Man from Mars)
Written on the back of the photo

The Soviet Union, not an official participant in the Korean War, had over 72,000 military personnel in North Korea and hundreds of Soviet Air Force pilots who secretly flew combat missions in Russian planes camouflaged with North Korean or Chinese colors and markings. At first, the Soviet pilots were forbidden from speaking Russian on their radios, but that later changed. The U.S. Military and government knew the Soviets were intervening in combat and countered with U.S. and U.N. fighter jets, but kept the Soviet involvement a secret from the public.[56]

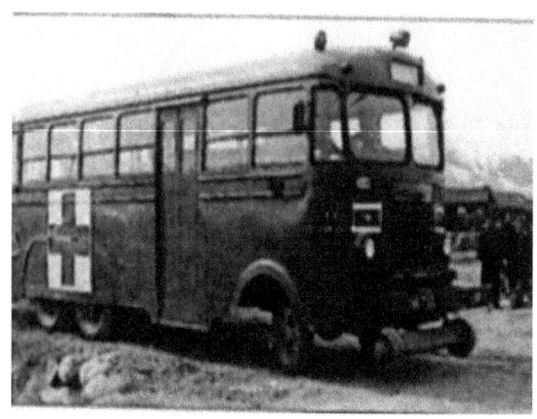

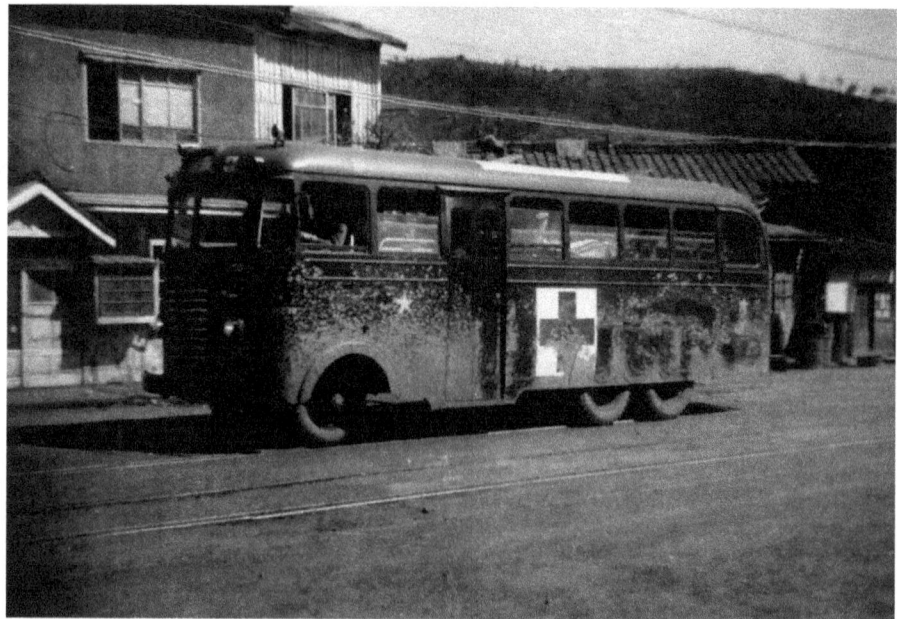

Litter bus used to transport patients from the hospital train to evacuation hospitals (two to four miles away.) Some of these buses were fitted with special rail wheels and served as rail ambulances to transport wounded from the evacuation hospitals to airfields when a hospital train was not available.
(Virginia Taylor's 1956 Stanford Thesis.)

(Photos courtesy of Virginia Taylor collection)

PRISONERS OF WAR (POW/PW)
Hospital Trains transported wounded POWs

Written in Chinese, this sign is telling the enemy of the good care they'd receive in U.S. hospitals and PW camps and offering safe conduct if they surrender.   (Courtesy of Virginia Taylor collection)

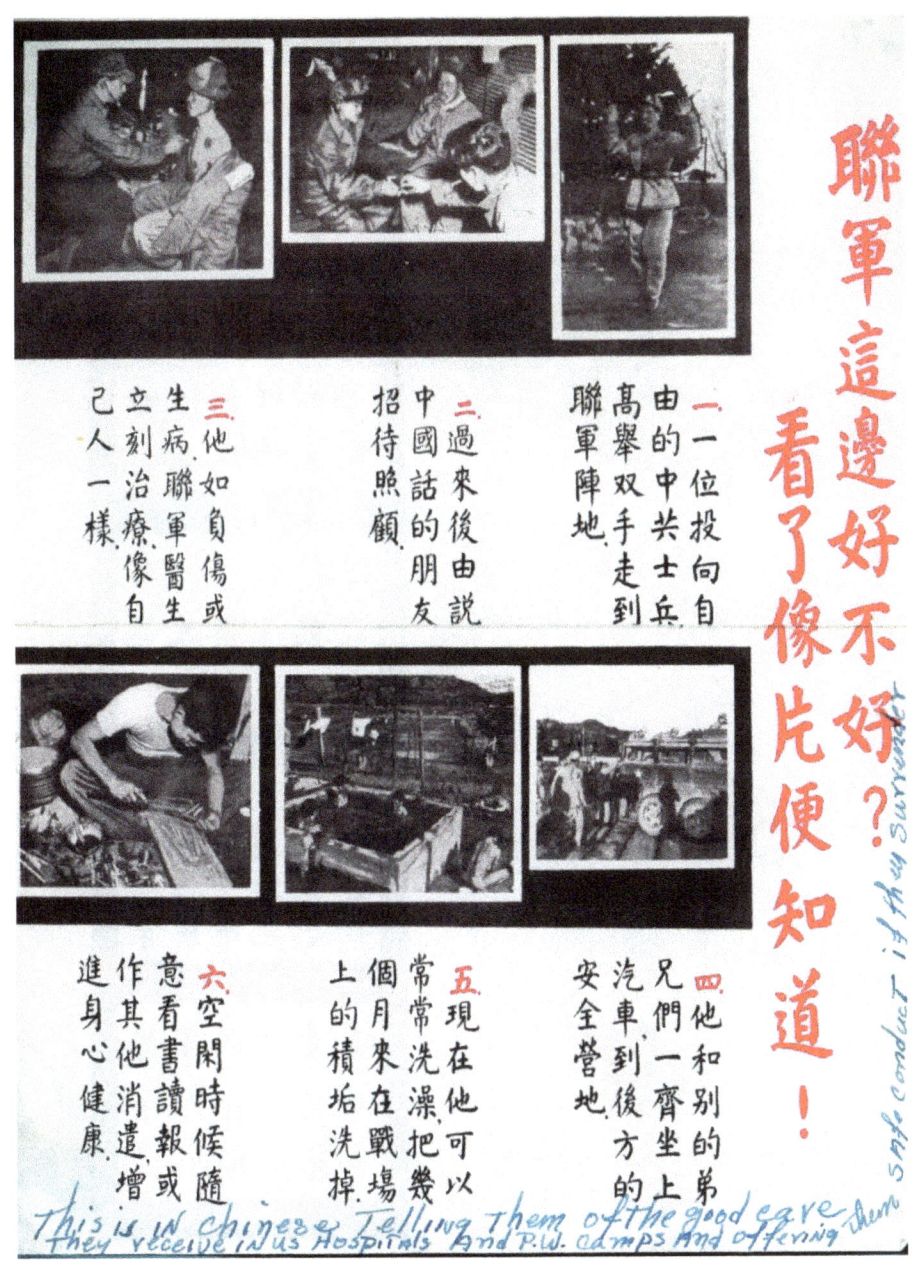

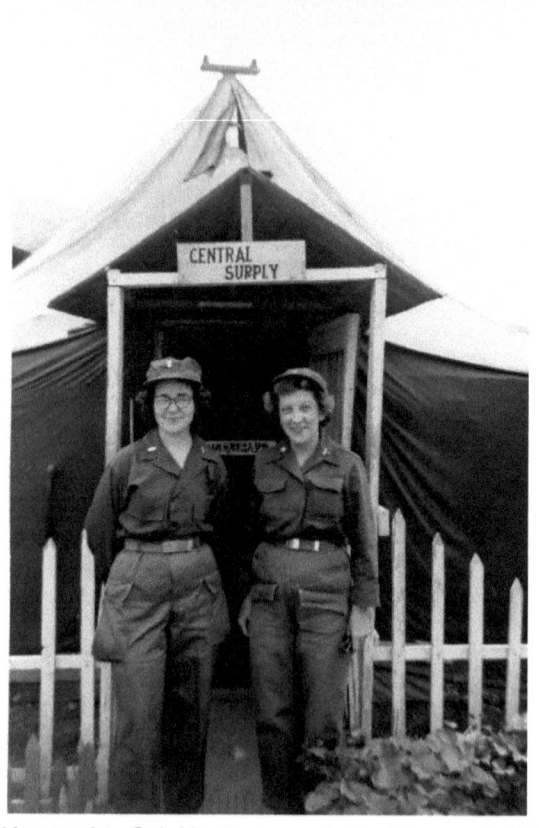

Nurses Lt. Sal Hardesty and Lt. Hagen at POW Hospital, Pusan. (Sal is one of Virginia's roommates at the 21st Evac Hospital.)

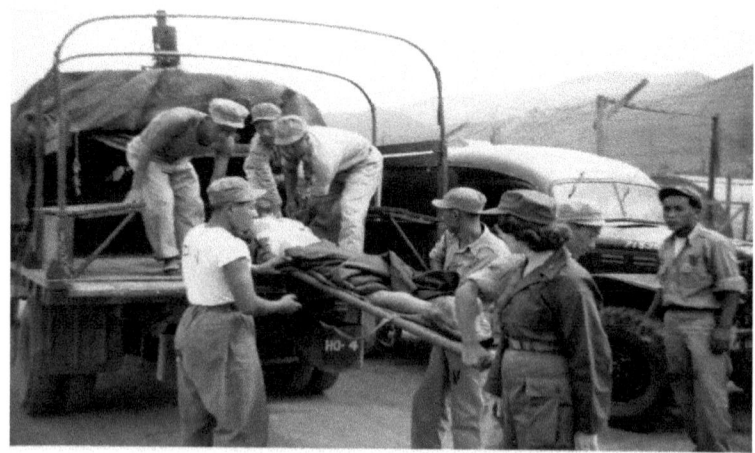

Sal supervises the unloading of the POWs to the POW hospital.

(Photos courtesy of Virginia Taylor collection)

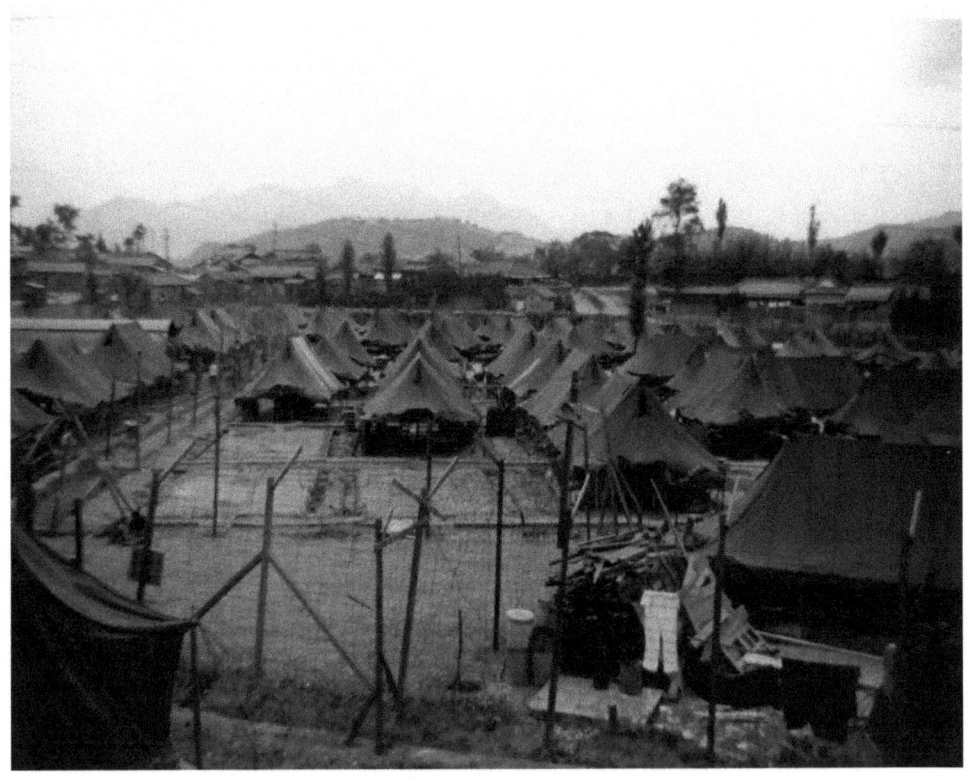

3rd and 14th Field convalescent POW Hospitals
(Photo courtesy of Virginia Taylor collection)

Staffed by American medical personnel, the prisoners got the best of medical care. The main hospital had the same type of equipment that was used on American wounded.

One section of the hospital was devoted to rehabilitation. Amputees were fitted with artificial limbs made by other prisoners with materials furnished by the United States. (Virginia Taylor's 1956 Stanford Thesis.)

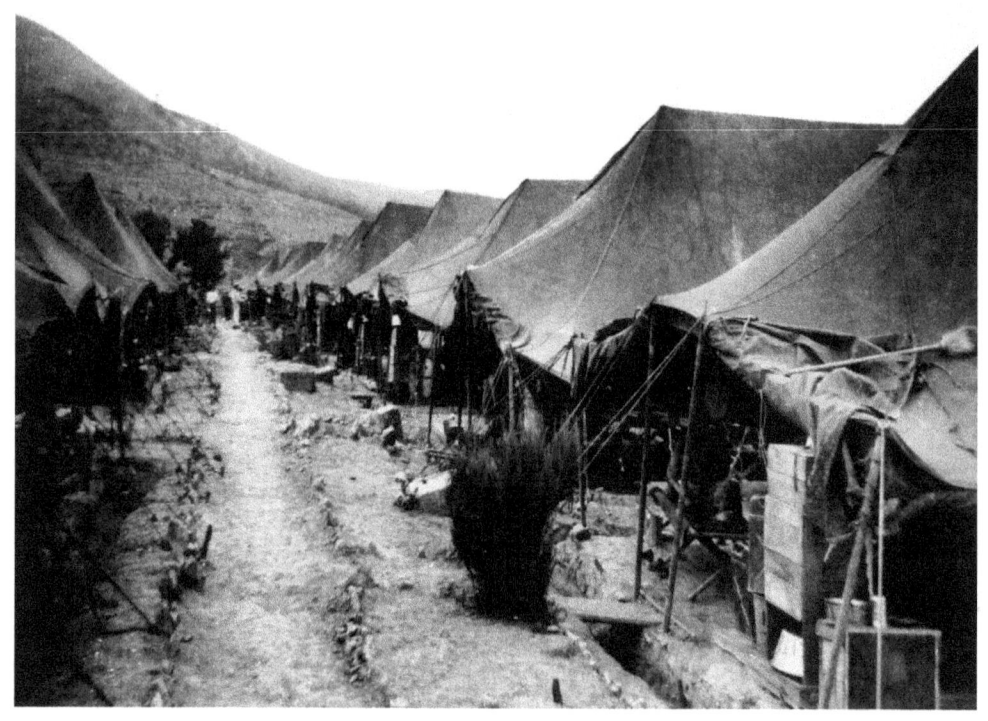

POW convalescent hospital, Pusan

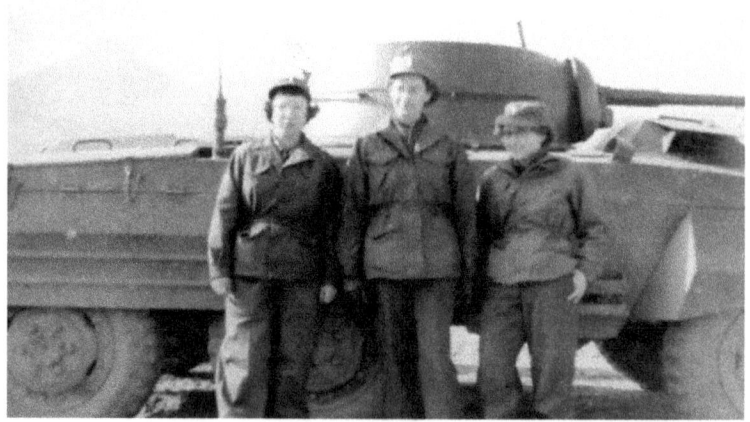

Lts Virginia Taylor and Evelyn Kropp with another nurse at the
14th Field POW convalescent Hospital

(Photos courtesy of Virginia Taylor collection)

North Korean Prisoner Tells All
Proj. 16-279, **14 January 1951**

"Before I entered the North Korean army, I was a businessman and a Communist. When the Russians entered North Korea, they put up many fine housing projects, hospitals, and made many jobs for Communist Party members. The rich were forced to give up their wealth and were sent to other provinces. The workers were organized into a People's Labor Party, were put into military uniform, trained by Russian soldiers, and sent into war against South Korea. When I saw that they were killing my people, I surrendered. Soviet Russia intends to dominate the whole world. Today I am convinced there are two ways of life, communism and democracy. The world must choose between them."[58]

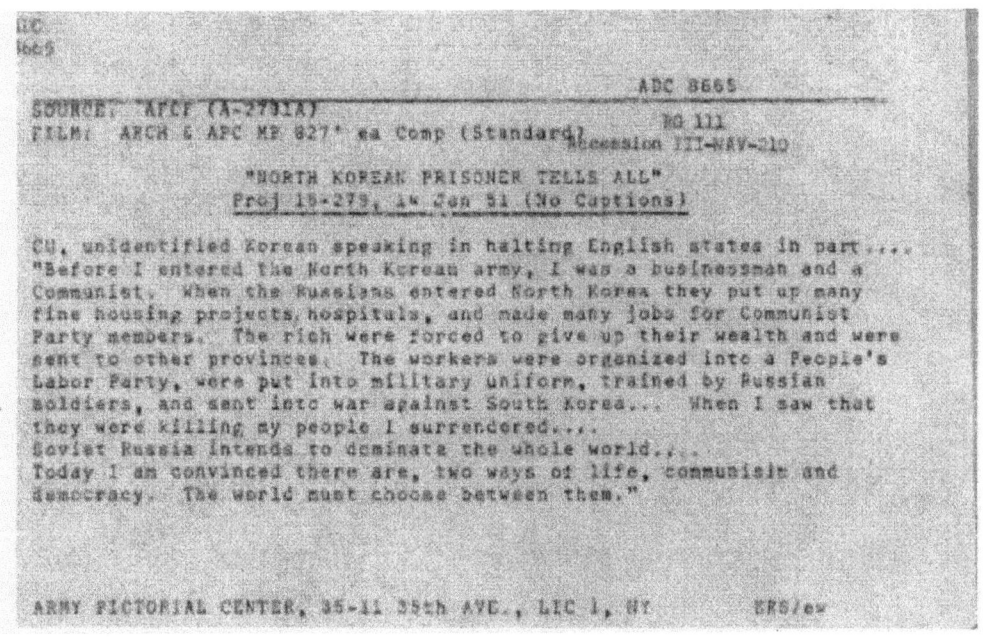

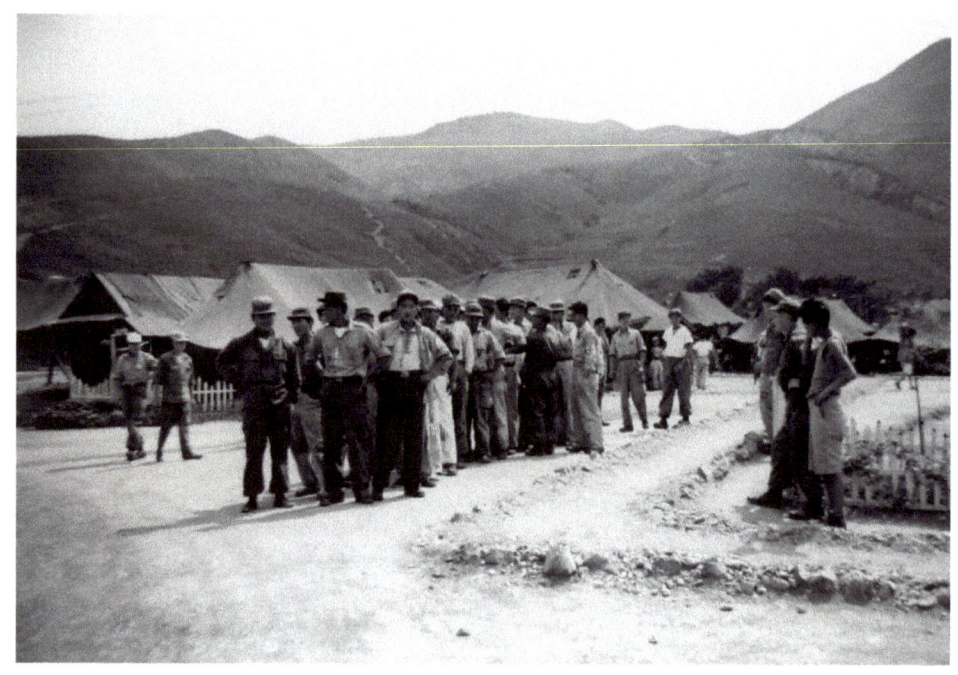

North Korean and Chinese POWs
Pusan, Korea

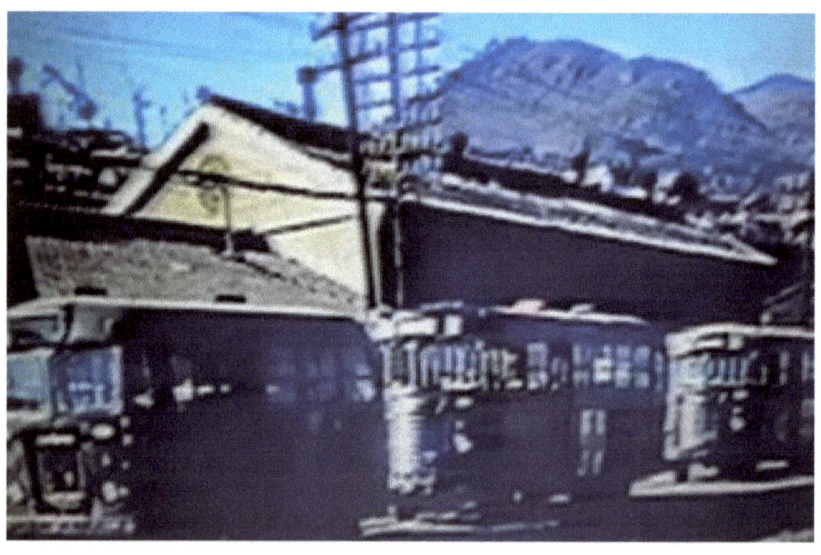

(Photos courtesy of Virginia Taylor collection)

OPERATION LITTLE SWITCH

In 1953 Panmunjom, North Korea, international changes began to register with breakthroughs toward peace. Under the new administration of President Eisenhower, the United States warned of severe consequences, including nuclear weapons. The death of Joseph Stalin in March signaled a power struggle in the Soviet Union. The burden of the Korean War was one that neither party wished to bear any longer, except for some of the Koreans themselves.[59]

On March 28, 1953, the Chinese and North Koreans agreed to U.N. proposals for the exchange of sick and wounded POWs. Finalized on April 11, 1953, the United Nations was to return 700 Chinese and 5,100 Koreans, or 4.5% of the 132,000 prisoners they held in custody. The Communists 450 South Koreans and 150 non-Korean POWs, or 5% of the 12,000 they held. The agreement provided for the exchange to take place at Panmunjom and allowed the Communists to move the wounded to the front in well-marked convoys over designated routes.[60] This first exchange was called Operation Little Switch (April 20-May 3, 1953).

The movement of Communist POWs to Panmunjom was a noisy affair. Demonstrations broke out at the camps. Prisoners riding from the island camps of Koje-do (a 150-square-mile island 20 miles off the southwestern coast of Korea) to the landing craft for transport to the mainland, threw away their rations of soap and tooth powder and tossed away cigarette packs containing hand-printed messages accusing the U.N. Command of "barbarous acts." Some went on hunger strikes; many mutilated their clothing to make themselves look maltreated.[61]

Updated numbers from Koreawar.org/history: The U.N. returned 1,030 Chinese and 5,194 Koreans. The Communist repatriated 684 U.N. sick and wounded.

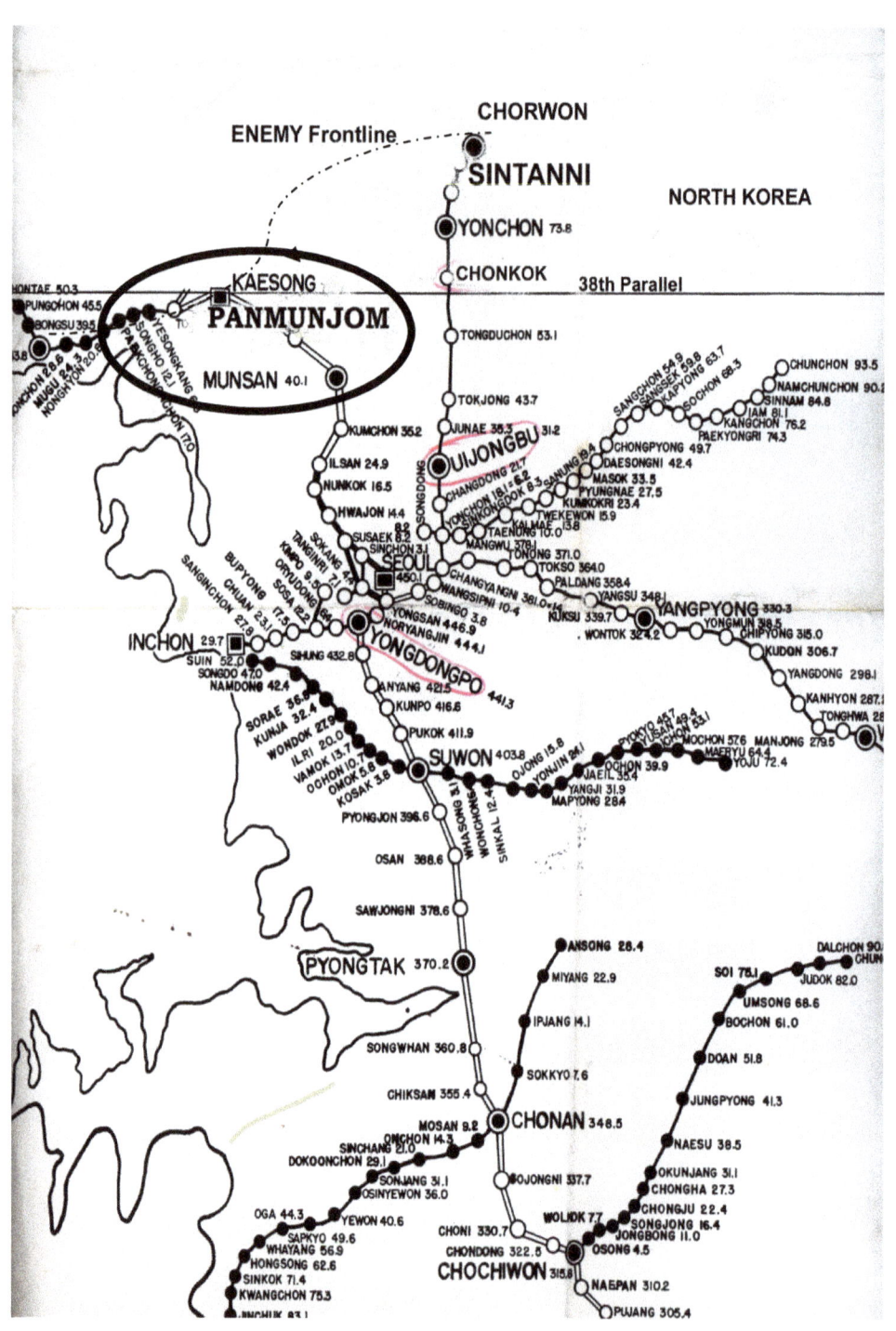

DON VERSTRAETE'S RECOLLECTION

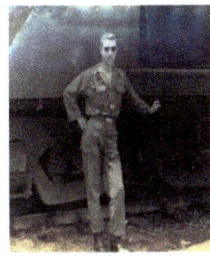

(Medic/Car Commander Train 106)

One week prior to April 20, 1953, **Hospital Train 106** was called out from Yongdongpo for a dry run of the prisoner exchange, *Operation Little Switch*. Except for the crew, the train traveled empty from Yongdongpo to Panmunjom, North Korea. Once there, the North Koreans and Swedish Red Cross toured the train. During the tour, the crew remained aboard, and shortly after, headed back to Yongdongpo.

PREPARATION (per military archives):
- The hospital cars were specially equipped with telephones for intra-train communication.
- Windows were covered with strong screens to protect passengers from rocks and other objects.
- The 3rd TMRS sent a pilot locomotive ahead for possible obstructions on the track.
- A wreck train equipped with a wrecking crane followed in case of derailment.
- The rules of the exchange: Every Train HAD to arrive on schedule.

APRIL 20, 1953:

- All eight hospital trains were used for Operation Little Switch, but left at separate times.
- The POWs were loaded in the hospital trains at the Pusan dock.
- Train 106 loaded EIGHTY North Korean POWs per car. (There were six cars per train.)

- In Don's car, the POWs lined each side of the lower bunks, sitting shoulder to shoulder.
- Train 106 departed mid-morning and arrived in Panmunjom early morning the next day.
- The train stopped twice for ice for the air conditioners. At each stop, armed soldiers lined both sides of the platforms.
- Throughout the trip, the POWs chanted for hours, ending with three fist pumps, hollering "Bonsai" after each pump. They'd rest a bit and start chanting again.
- One POW insisted on visiting the other cars. The interpreter talked to him. Ultimately, the POW was refused.
- The vestibule was crammed with the medics/corpsman plus two MPs per car.
- The mood was complacent.
- None of the crew interacted with the POWs. No meals were served.
- No sleep by any of the crew.
- Once the train stopped in Panmunjom, the POWs were offered a clear broth by the Swedish Red Cross. All refused.
- The Swedish Red Cross assisted the North Koreans with the POW transfer.
- None of the crew got off the train.

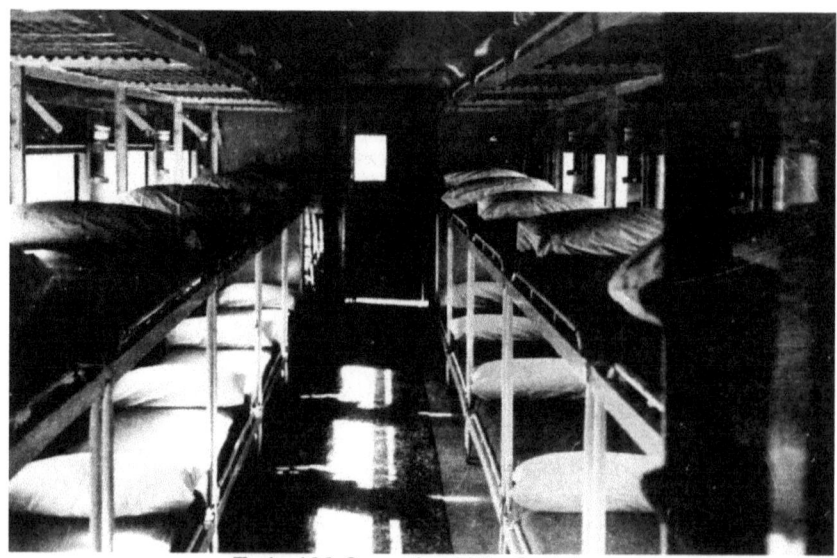

Train 106 Operation Little Switch
Eighty POWs in one Hospital Unit Car

(Photo courtesy of Virginia Taylor collection)

COLOR SLIDES
Taken with Virginia Taylor's new camera

Excerpt of Virginia Taylor February 1952 letter:
I have bought me a 35mm camera, which takes <u>color slide pictures</u> as well as black and whites. Will send a viewer and my boxes of slides as I take them and you will get a better picture of what the place is really like.

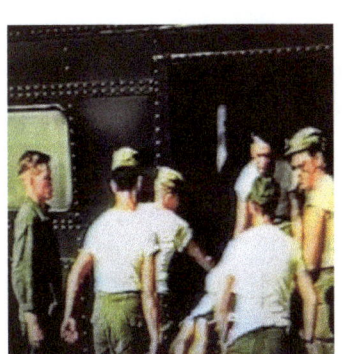
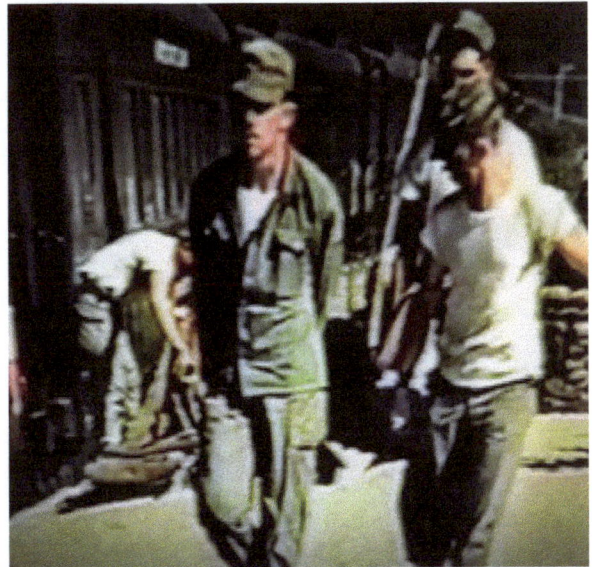

Train 105 medics loading wounded

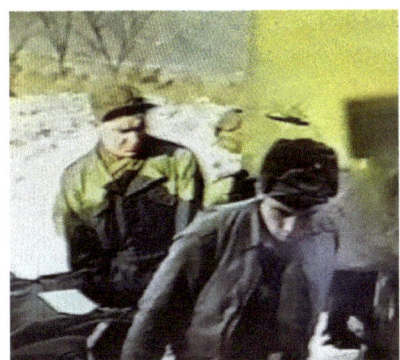

Snow-covered ground
Medics loading wounded

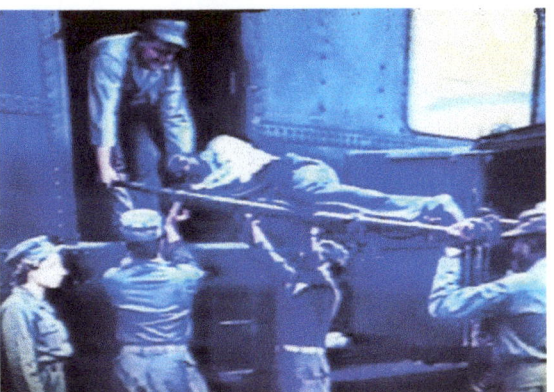

Medics loading <u>Turkish soldier</u> onto the hospital train

(Photos courtesy Virginia Taylor collection)

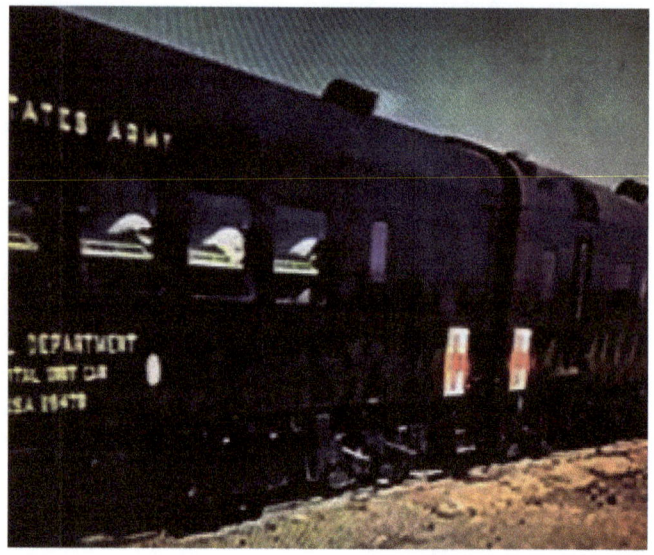

Hospital Unit Car 89478 (TRAIN 105)

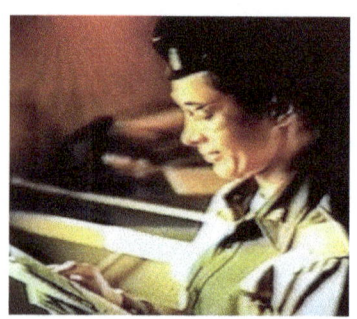 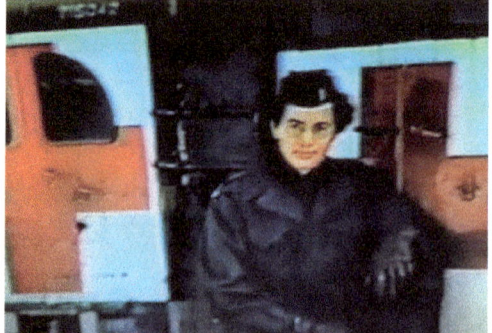

1st Lt. (Nurse) Virginia Taylor

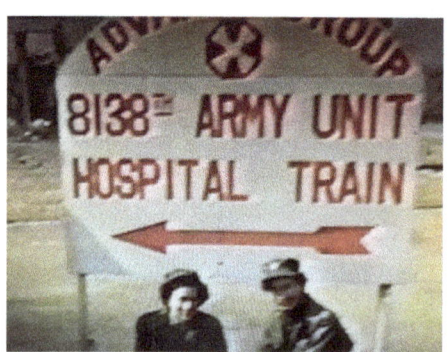 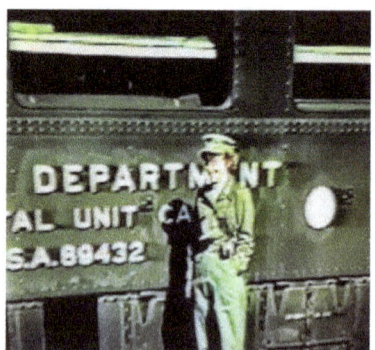

Betty Potocik and Virginia Taylor

1st Lt. (Nurse) Evelyn Kropp
(TRAIN 102)

(Photos courtesy Virginia Taylor collection)

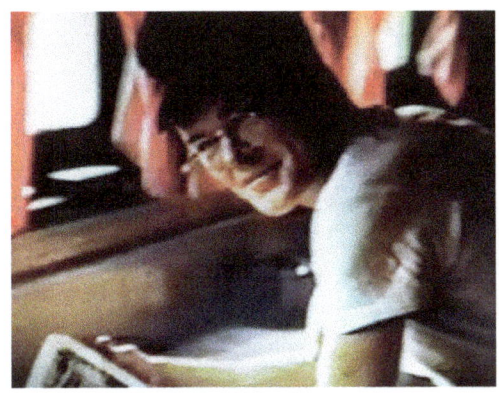

Mess Sergeant/Chief Cook
Lloyd Englebyecht
(TRAIN 105)

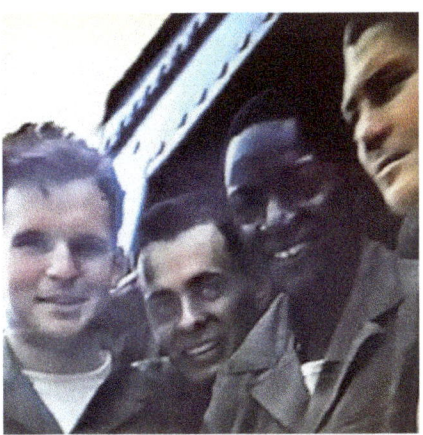

Train 105 Medics/Crew

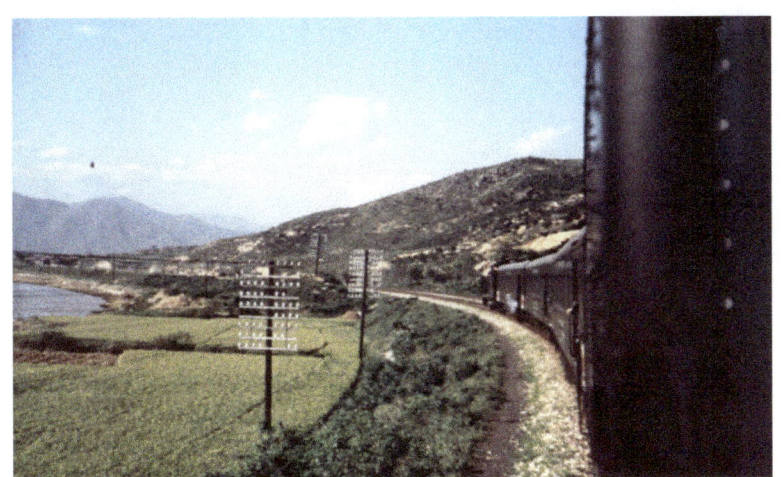

TRAIN 105
(Photos courtesy of Virginia Taylor collection)

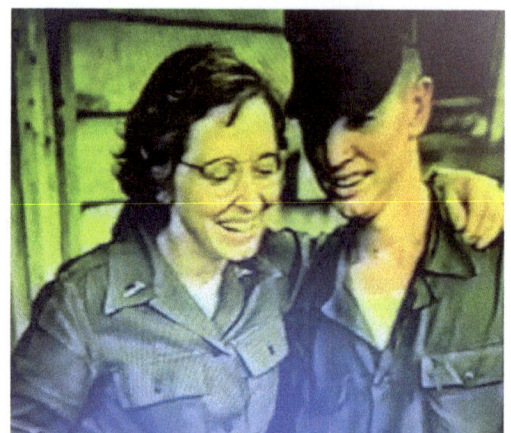

21st Evac Nurse Evelyn Kropp with Crew Chief Anderson

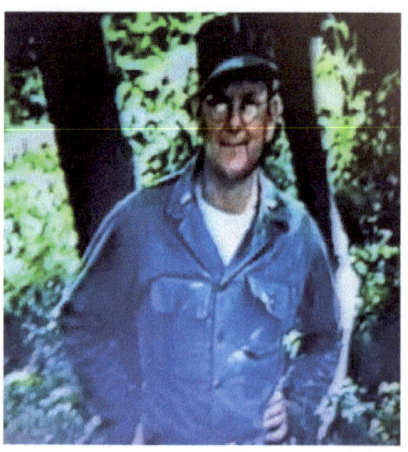

DOC Bauer

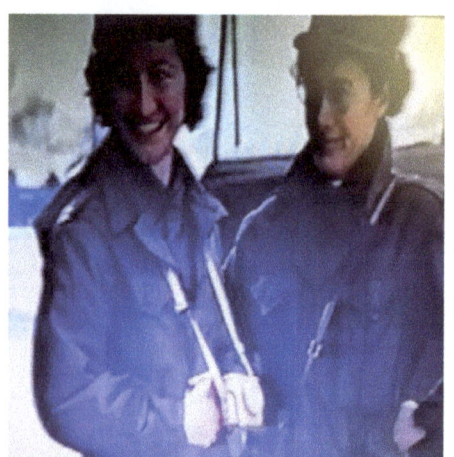

Train Nurses: Capt. Lena Toole and Lt. Virginia Taylor

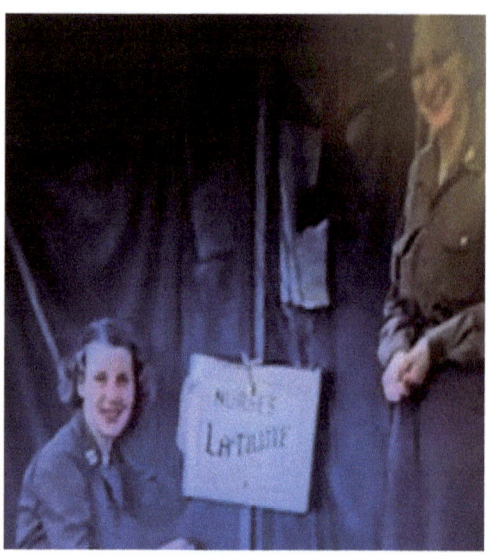

8055 MASH Nurses
SIGN: Nurses LATRINE

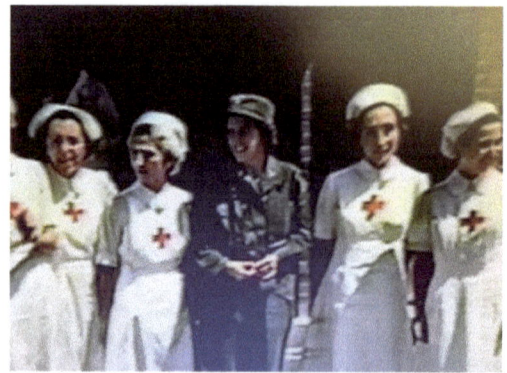

Capt. Lundstrum (Pinky) Chief Nurse Swedish Hospital and Swedish Red Cross Nurses

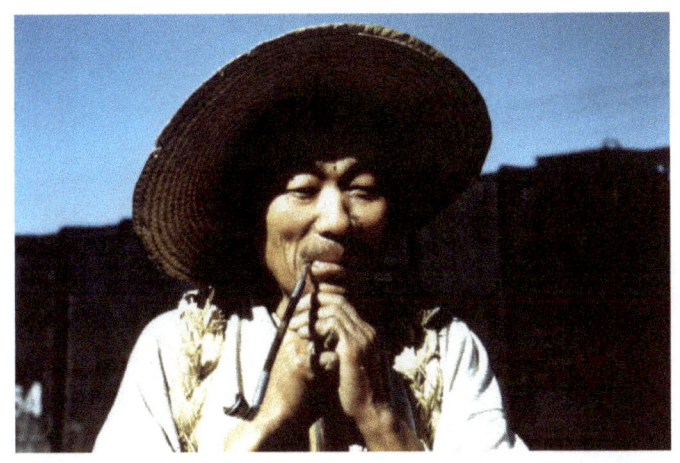

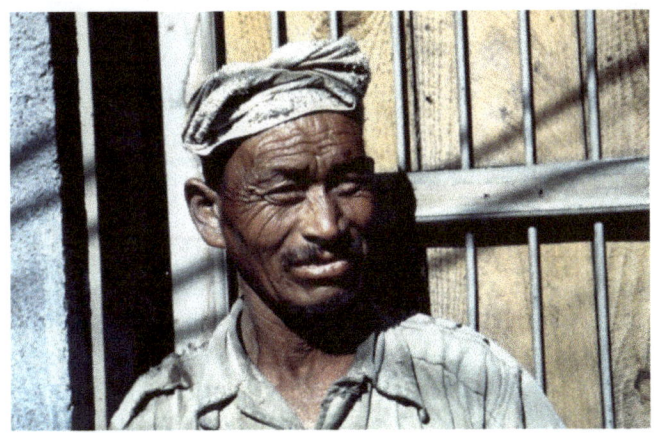

PAPASANS
(Photos courtesy of
Virginia Taylor
collections)

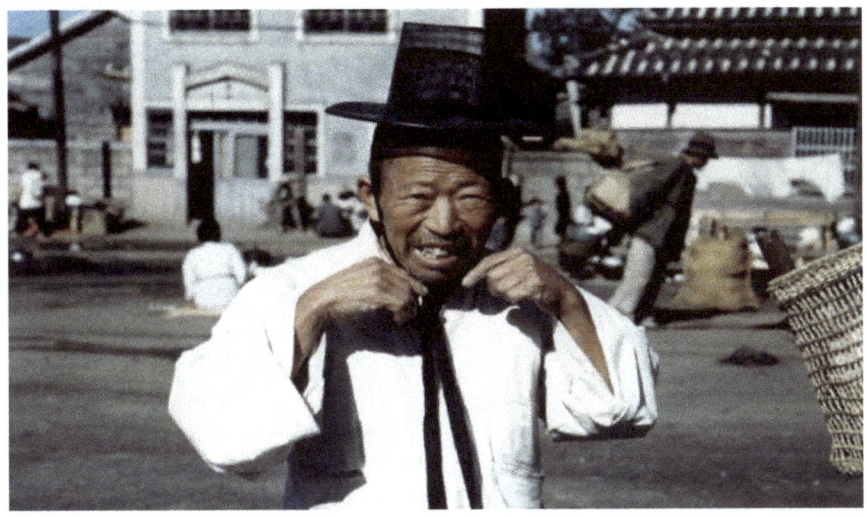

 Lt. Virginia Taylor's
EIGHTH UNITED
STATES ARMY
(EUSA)
Shoulder Sleeve
Insignia

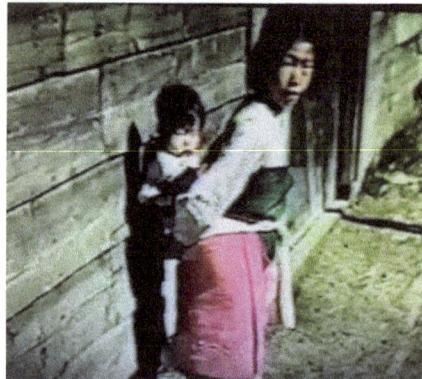

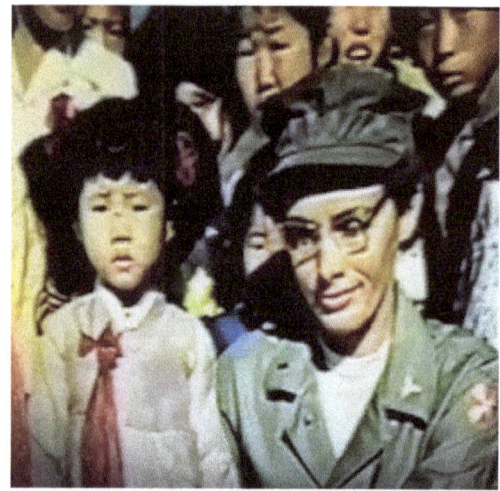

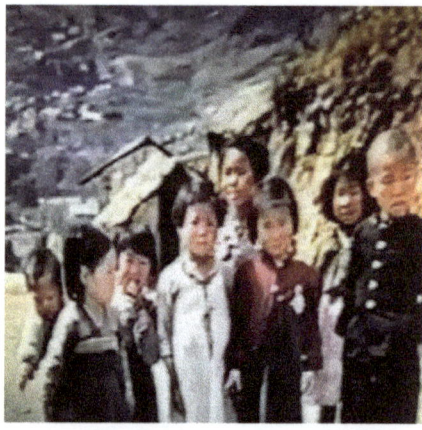

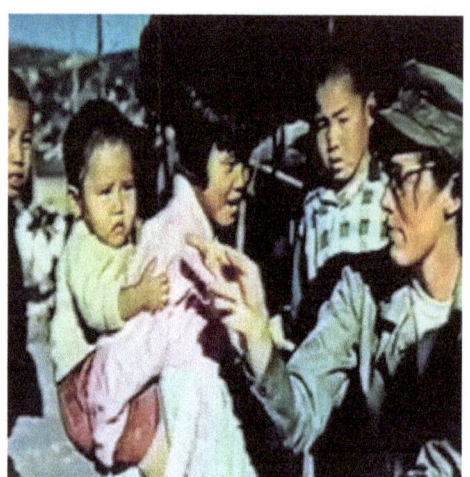

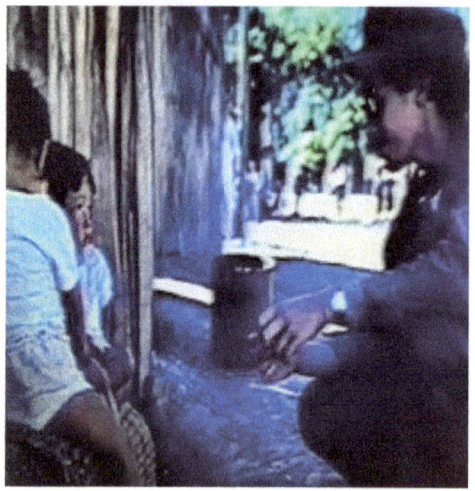

(Photos courtesy of Virginia Taylor collection)

NORTH KOREA WAR ZONE

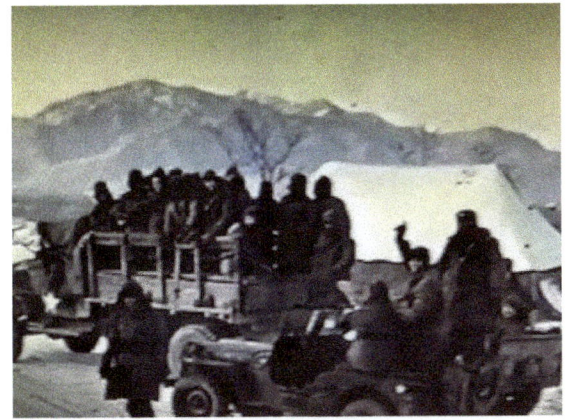
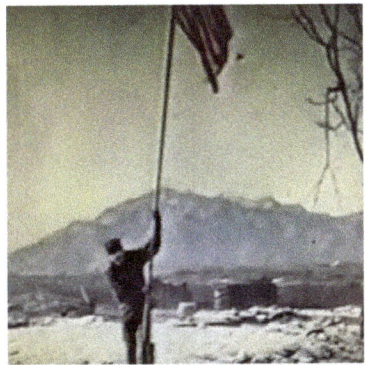

Our boys heading to the frontline

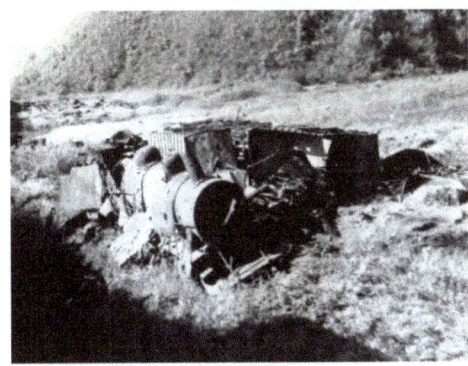

Blown up locomotive NORTH KOREA

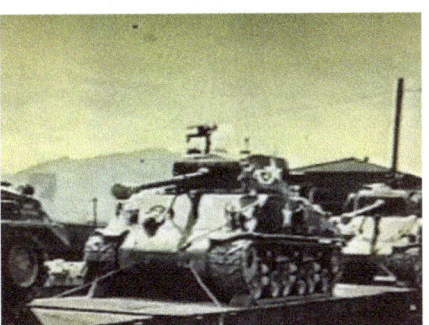

More tanks arriving from the States

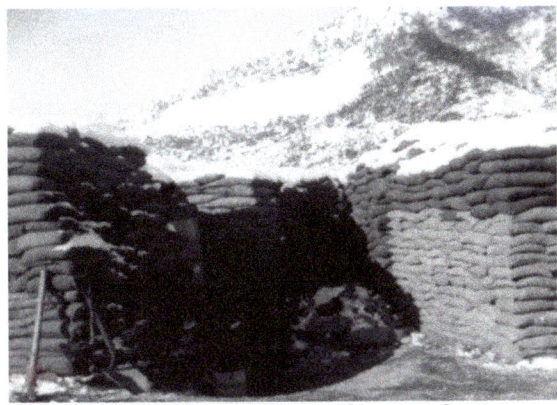

Sandbag barrier at Sintanni Clearing Station
NORTH KOREA

(Photos courtesy of Virginia Taylor collection)

NORTH KOREA WAR ZONE
SINTANNI CLEARING STATION 8,000 YARDS FROM ENEMY FRONTLINES

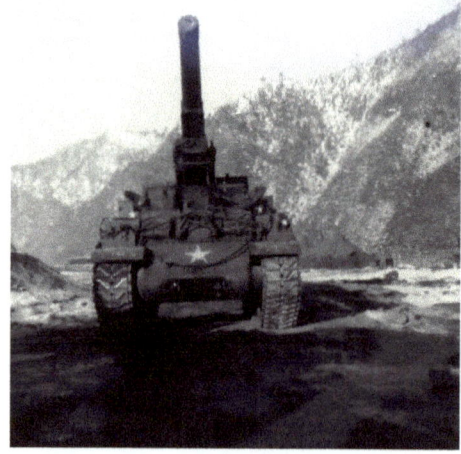

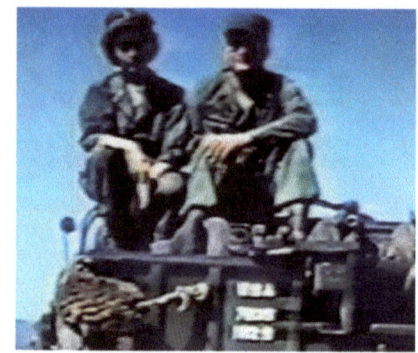

Virginia and train doctor

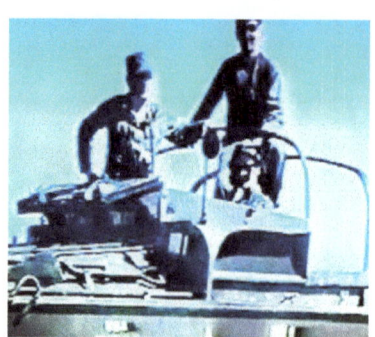

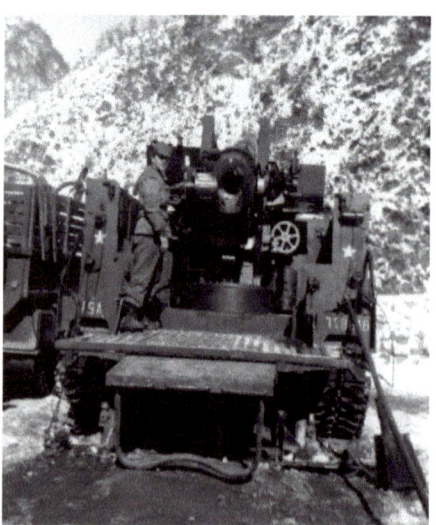

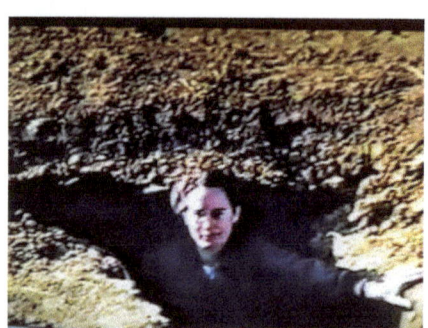

(Photos courtesy of Virginia Taylor collection)

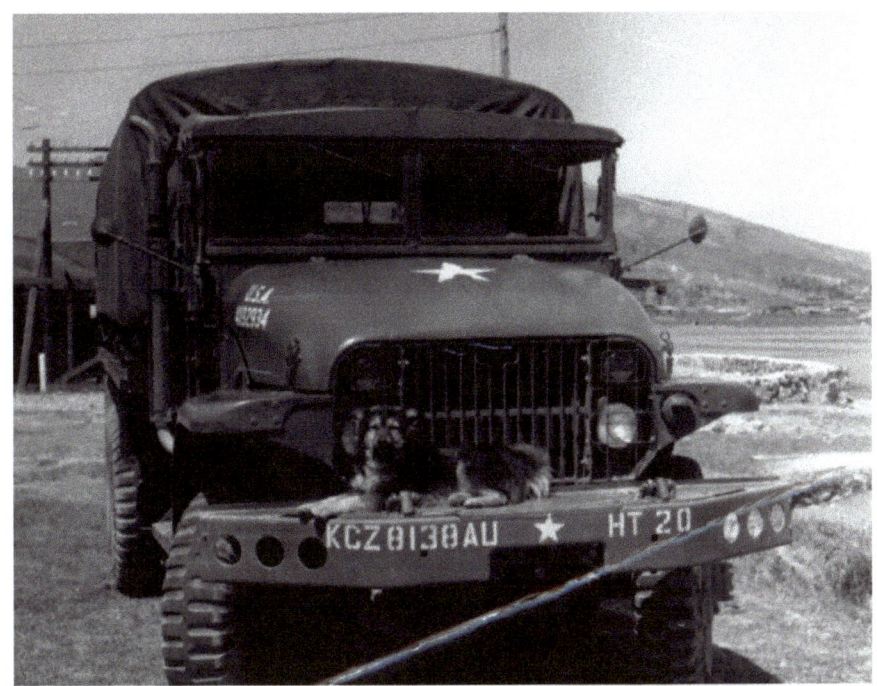

(Photo courtesy of Don Verstraete collection)
Note the dog on the front bumper

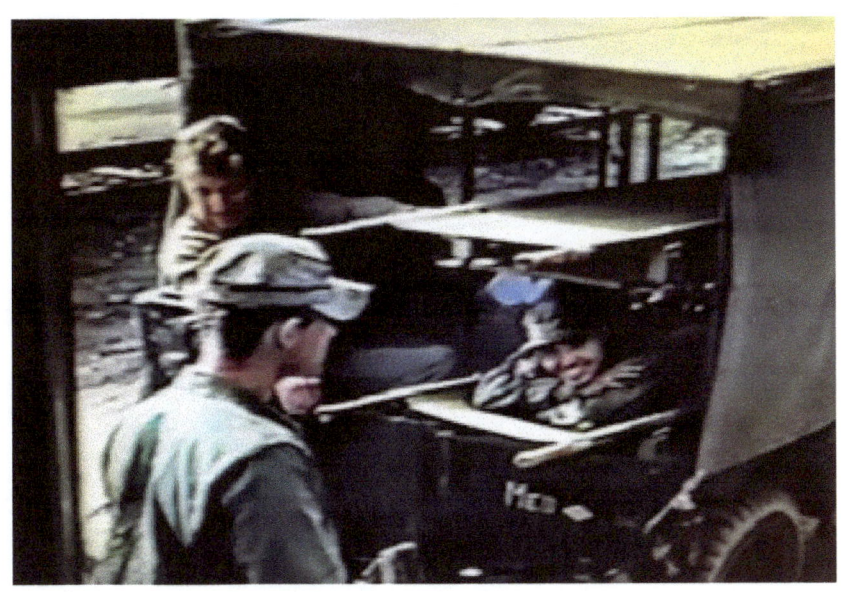

(Photo courtesy of Virginia Taylor collection)

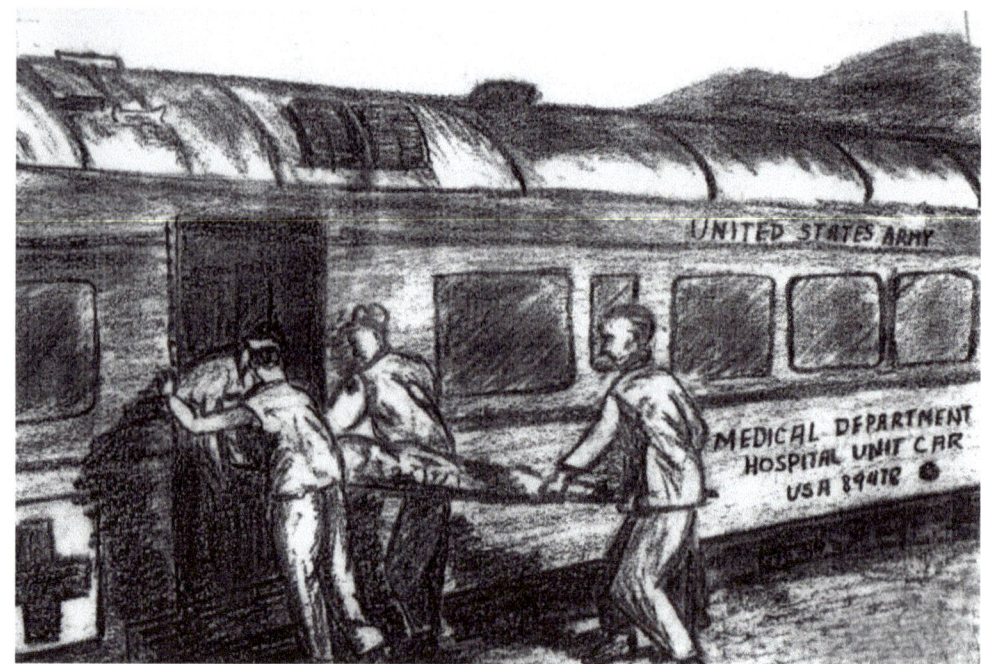

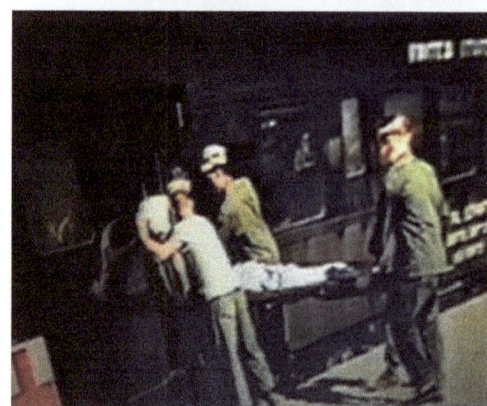

Sketch drawn for Virginia's 1956's Stanford Thesis from this picture.

Hospital car 89478

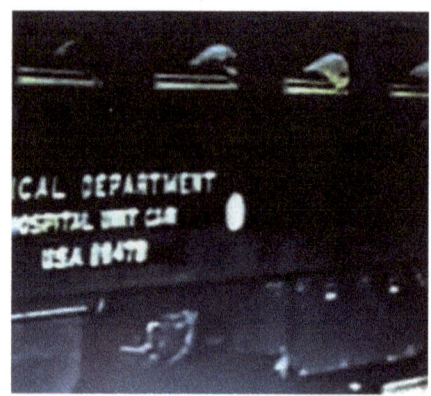

U.N. NURSES CONFERENCE

More than sixty nurses representing eight U.N. countries were in attendance at the association meeting held at 121st EVAC Hospital, Yongdongpo, Korea. July 1952

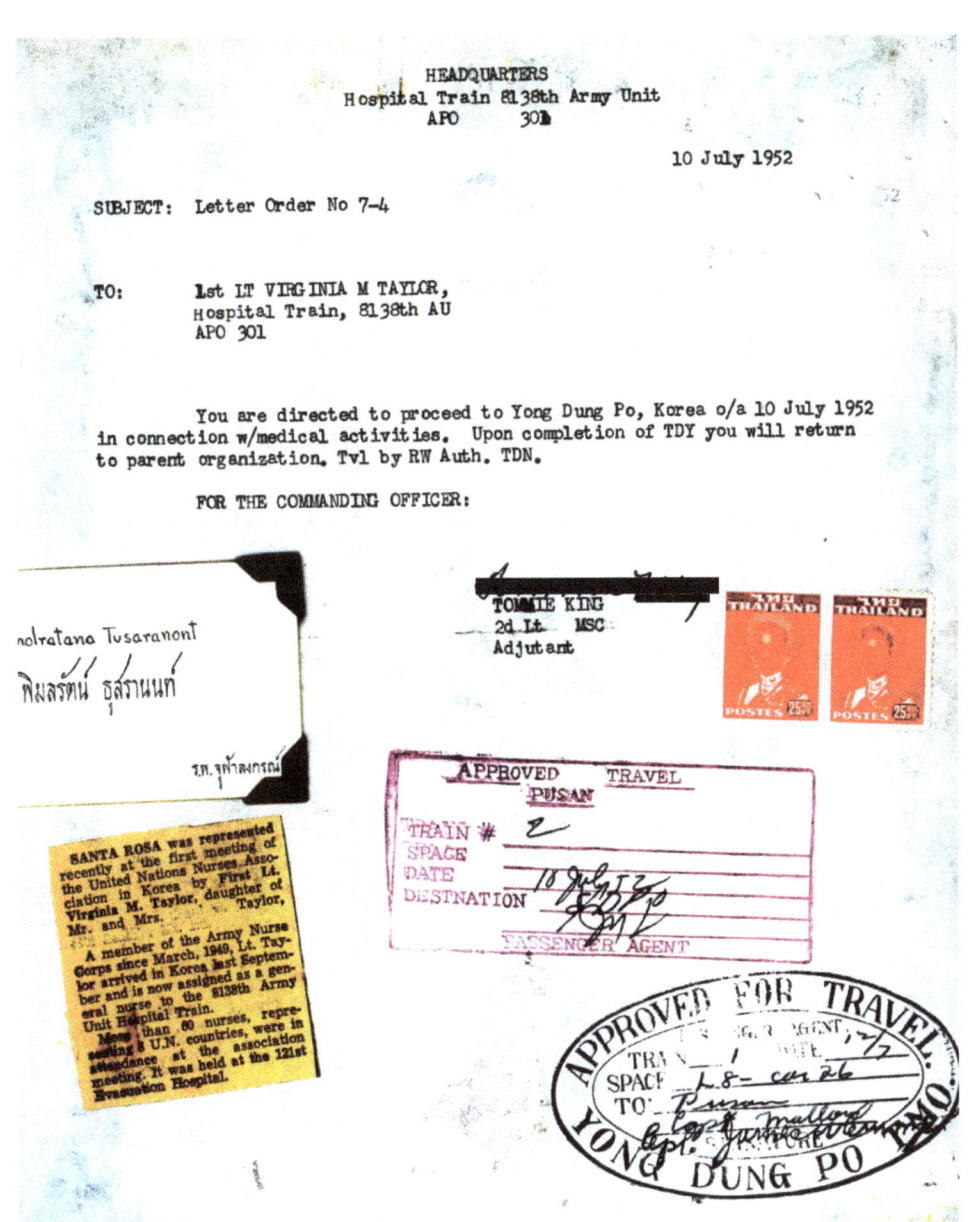

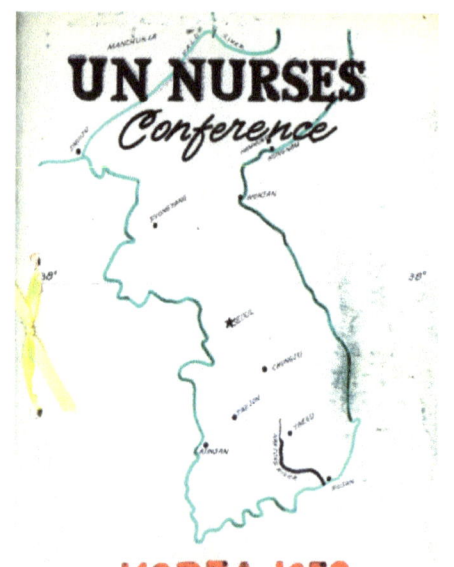

KOREA 1952

(Photos courtesy of Virginia Taylor collection)

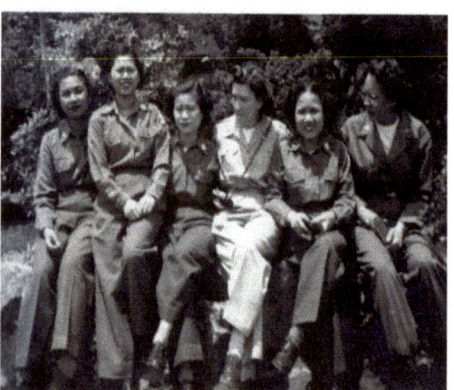

Lt. Betty Potocik and Lt. Virginia Taylor with Thailand Nurses

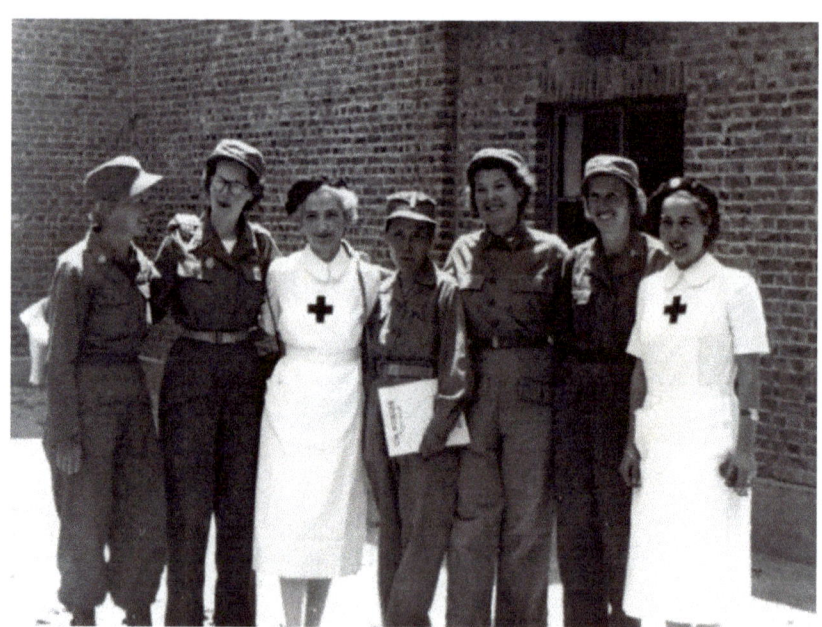

<u>2nd from Left</u>: Maj. Eunice Coleman
<u>In white</u>: Red Cross Italian Nurses
<u>2nd from Right</u>: Lt. Lundstrum (Pinky) the Swedish Hospital Chief Nurse

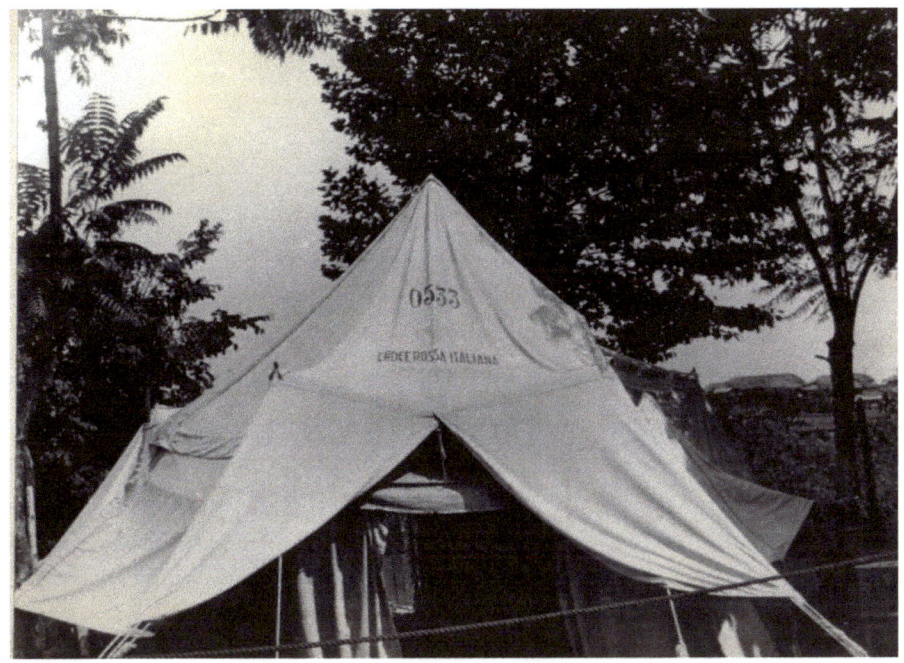

ITALIAN RED CROSS

ITALIAN RED CROSS HOSPITAL #68 (YONGDONGPO) arrived in Korea November 1951 with six nurses, seven doctors, twenty corpsmen. (All volunteers). The main building is located in an old school building with 150-bed capacity. The Medical and Surgical Dispensaries and a Tuberculosis clinic were held in tents like this one. (Virginia Taylor 1956 Stanford thesis)

(Photos courtesy of Virginia Taylor collection)

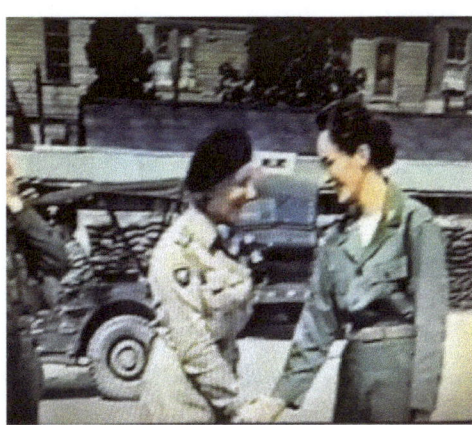

Lt. VirginiaTaylor and Italian Red Cross Chief Nurse

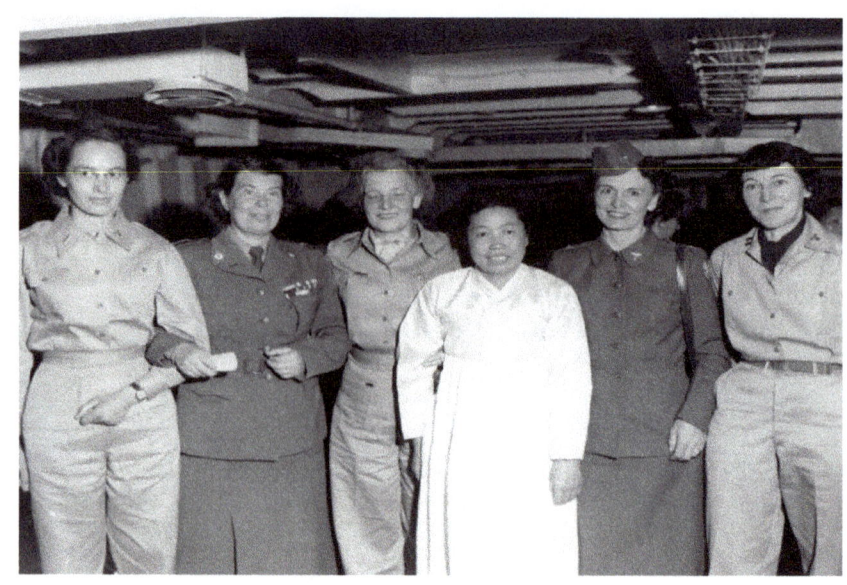

FLORENCE NIGHTINGALE BANQUET (MAY 1952) PUSAN

LtoR: Lt. Virginia Taylor (U.S.), Maj Nilson (Sweden) Lt. Koopman (Netherlands), Mus. Pok Soon Kong (Pusan), Capt. Browning (U.S.), Capt. Hanion (U.S.) 21st EVAC Hospital

(Photos courtesy of Virginia Taylor collection)

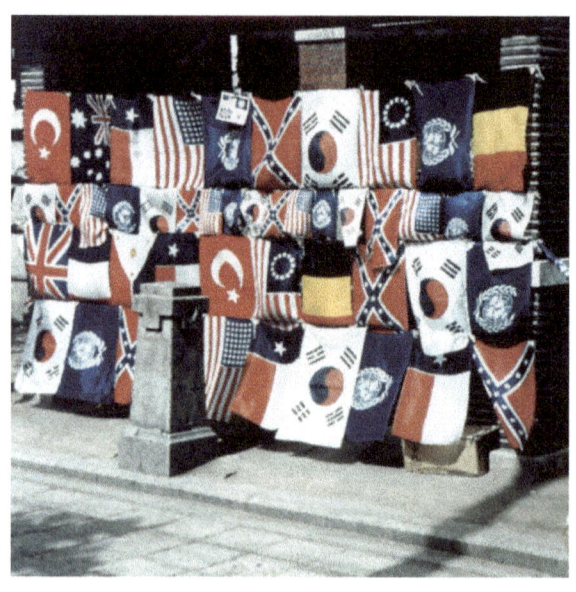

LASTING FRIENDSHIPS
MAJ. EUNICE COLEMAN
Bronze Star

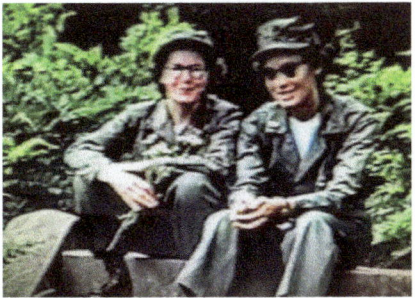

Eunice and Virginia

October 3, 1950 at three a.m., Maj. Eunice Coleman headed a motor convoy of twelve nurses from Inchon to Pusan under escort of soldiers. As machine-gun bullets whizzed overhead, she gathered her nurses in a ditch and outlined a course of action to care for the wounded as soon as they could feasibly reach them. She was decorated with the Bronze Star in February 1951. Lt. General Ridgway, Lt. General Almond, and Maj. General Ruffner were in attendance. She served in World War II and the Korean War. Her niece Nancy stated that Eunice loved the Army and was proud to be part of it. She passed away in 1983 at the age of 80 in Los Angeles, California.

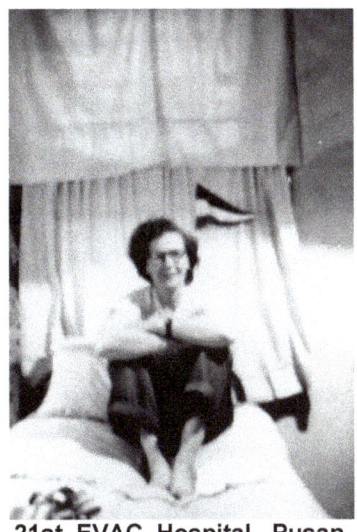

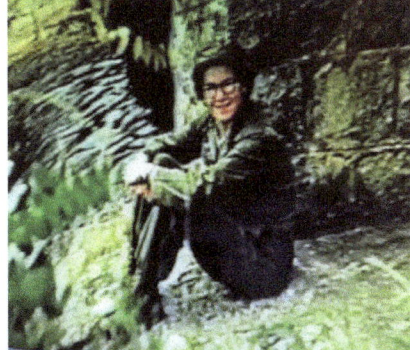

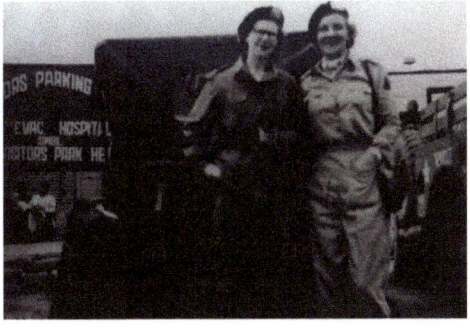

21st EVAC Hospital, Pusan, Korea (Photos courtesy of Virginia Taylor collection)

LT. SAL HARDESTY AND
LT. MASAKO NISHIYAMA (Nickey)
(Virginia's roommates at the 21st Evac Hospital, Pusan)

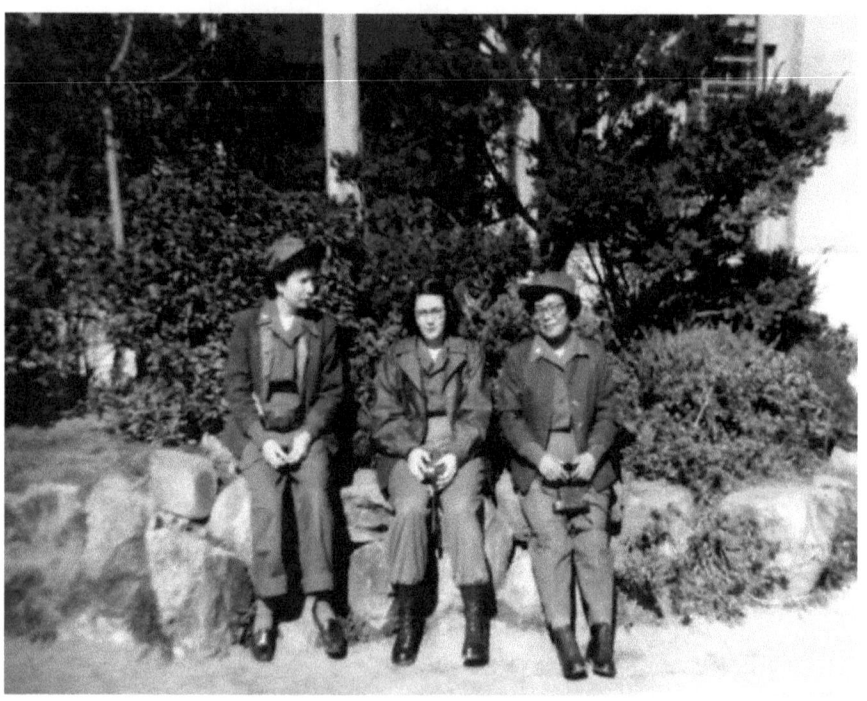

VIRGINIA'S THREE ROOMMATES: NURSES: Betty Potocik, Sal Hardesty, Masako Nishiyama (Nickey) (Photos courtesy of Virginia Taylor collection)

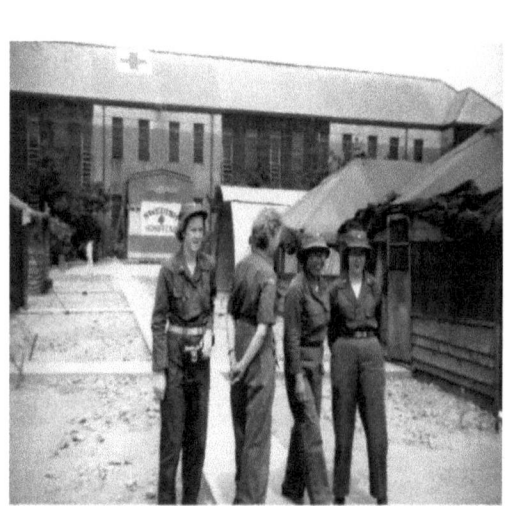

Nickey and Sal with Lt. Lundstrum, Chief Nurse of the Swedish Hospital

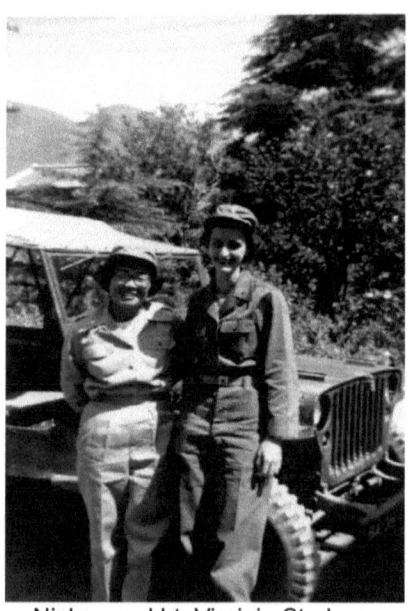

Nickey and Lt. Virginia Starkey

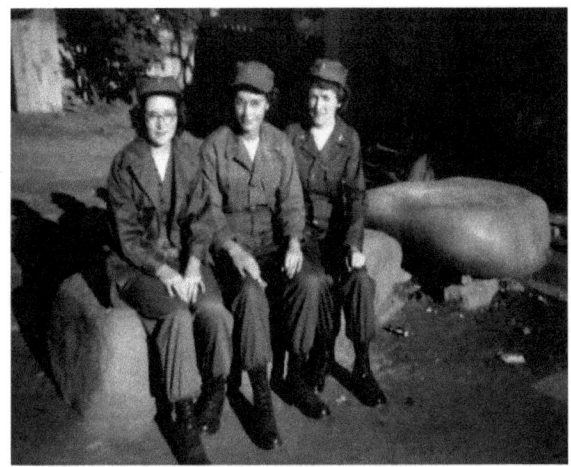

Sal, Virginia, and Lt. Sammons at the Maryknoll Sisters Convent, Pusan

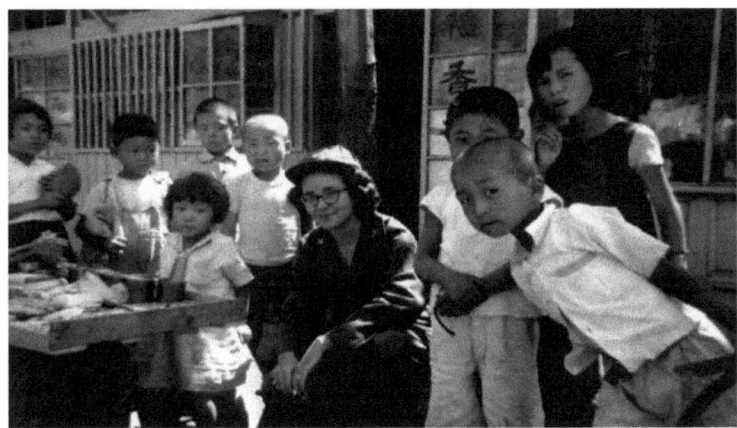

Sal with orphans

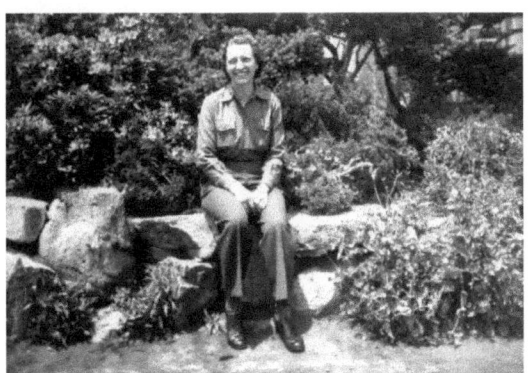

Captain Drack, Chief Nurse 21st Evac Hospital

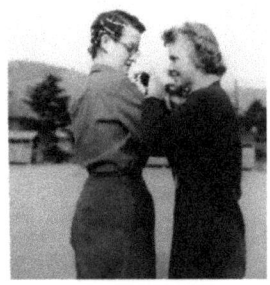

21st Evac nurses clowning around

LT. EVELYN KROPP

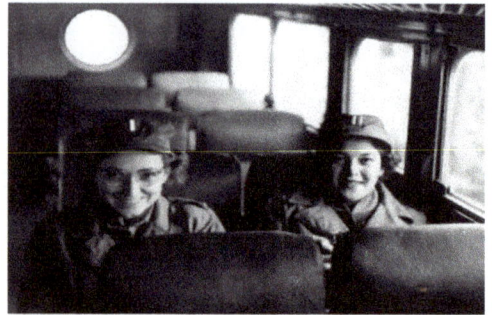

Evelyn with Corrine Bryant

(Photos courtesy of Virginia Taylor collection)

After basic training, Evelyn transferred to overseas duty at the Ryukyu Hospital, Okinawa. She later transferred to the 3rd Station Hospital (an old converted schoolhouse) in Pusan, Korea. While there, she served on the 8138th hospital train #102 as the only Medical Officer along with 10 enlisted men due to a shortage of doctors at that time. She loved the duty, but at five feet tall, she had difficulty reaching the top bunks so went back to hospital duty after two months.

In 1953, she discharged from the Army and began her career as a public health nurse for 25 years until her retirement in 1987. She passed away in 2019 at the Old Soldier's Home in Quincy, Illinois at the age of 95.

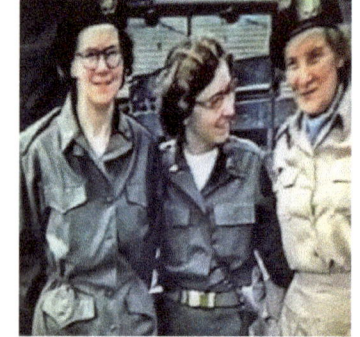

Evelyn with Eunice Coleman and the Italian (Red Cross) Chief Nurse

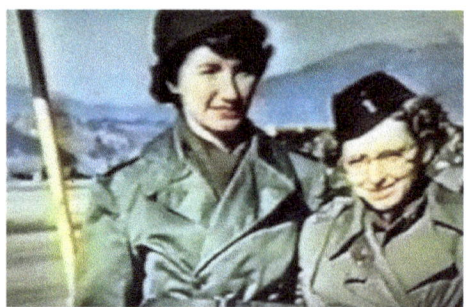

Train Nurse 108, Capt. Lena Toole and Evelyn at the airfield

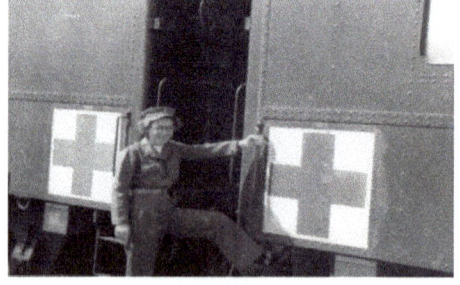

Evelyn (Train 102)

LT. ROSEMARY MAHONEY

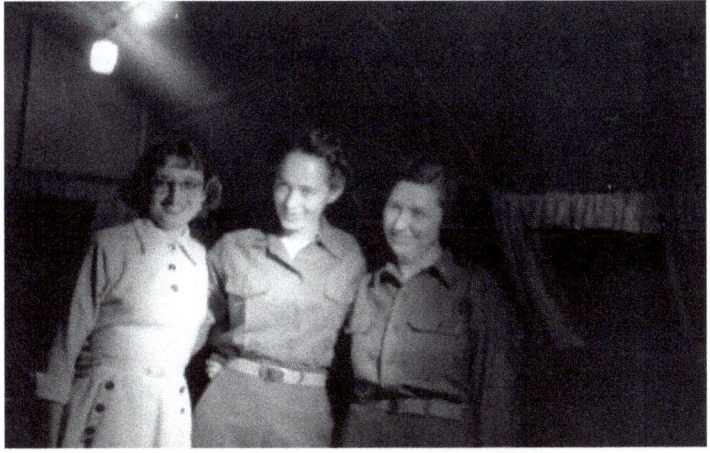

Rosemary, Virginia, Unknown nurse
Virginia's going away party (1953)

After Korea, Rosemary became a lifelong officer in the U.S. Army Nurse Corps. She retired as a Colonel in 1980 and served in Japan, Korea, Germany, Viet Nam, and the United States. She passed away in 2016 at the age of 87 and is buried at Arlington National Cemetery.

(Photos courtesy of Virginia Taylor collection)

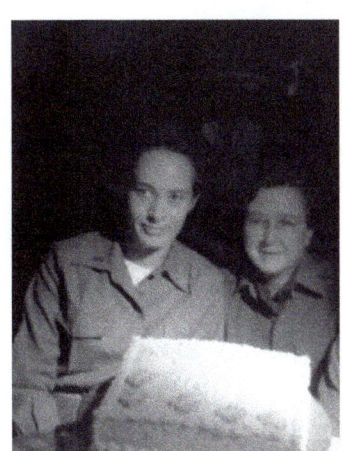

Virginia and Charlotte Lanternier (Train 104) at Virginia's going away party

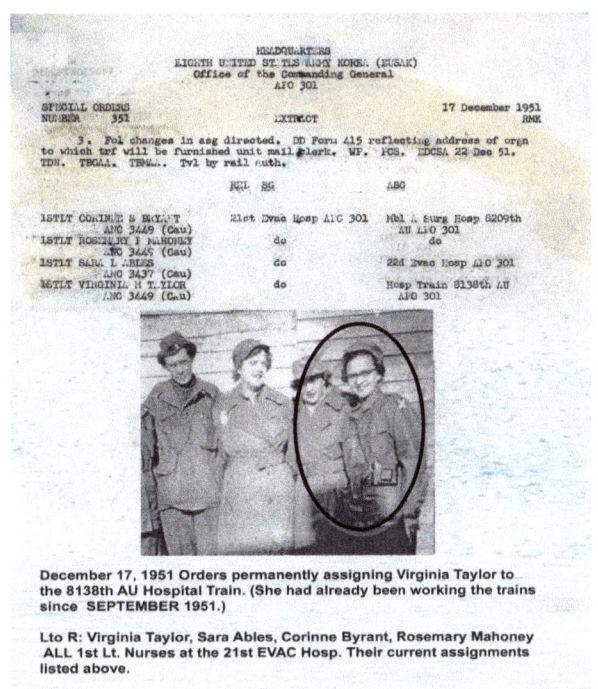

December 17, 1951 Orders permanently assigning Virginia Taylor to the 8138th AU Hospital Train. (She had already been working the trains since SEPTEMBER 1951.)

L to R: Virginia Taylor, Sara Ables, Corinne Byrant, Rosemary Mahoney ALL 1st Lt. Nurses at the 21st EVAC Hosp. Their current assignments listed above.

LT. BETTY (ELIZABETH) POTOCIK (Train 103)

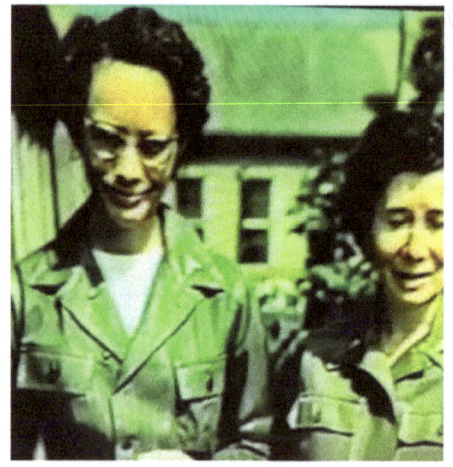
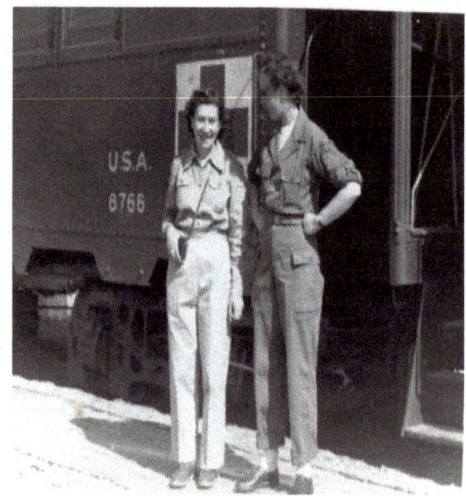

Virginia and Betty

After leaving Korea, Betty (Elizabeth) Potocik stationed at West point and remained in the U.S. Army Nurse Corps. She passed away at age 83 and is buried at the U.S. Military Academy Cemetery, West Point, NY.

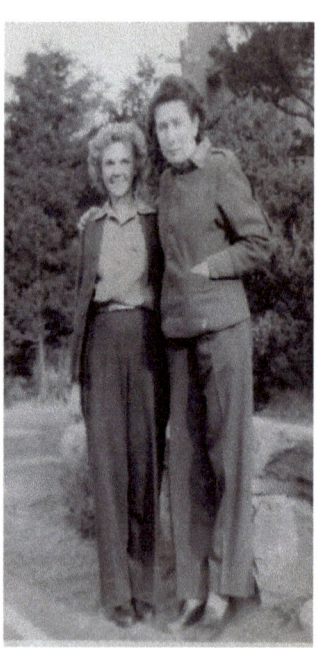

Betty and 21st EVAC nurse

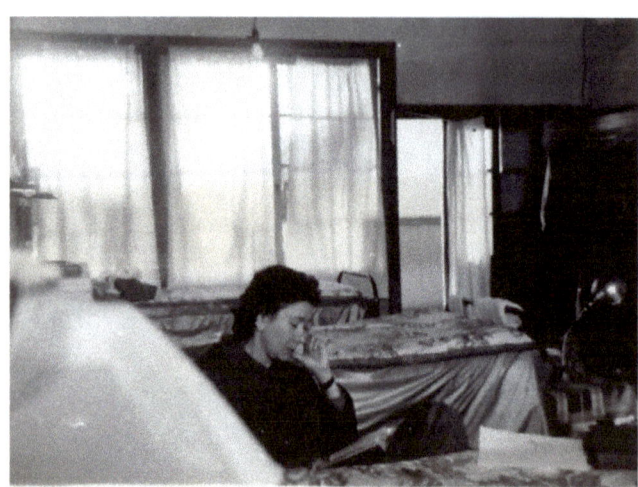

Betty at 21st EVAC Hospital, Pusan

(Photos courtesy of Virginia Taylor collection)

BANCHONG AKSORNINDRA (THAILAND RED CROSS NURSE)

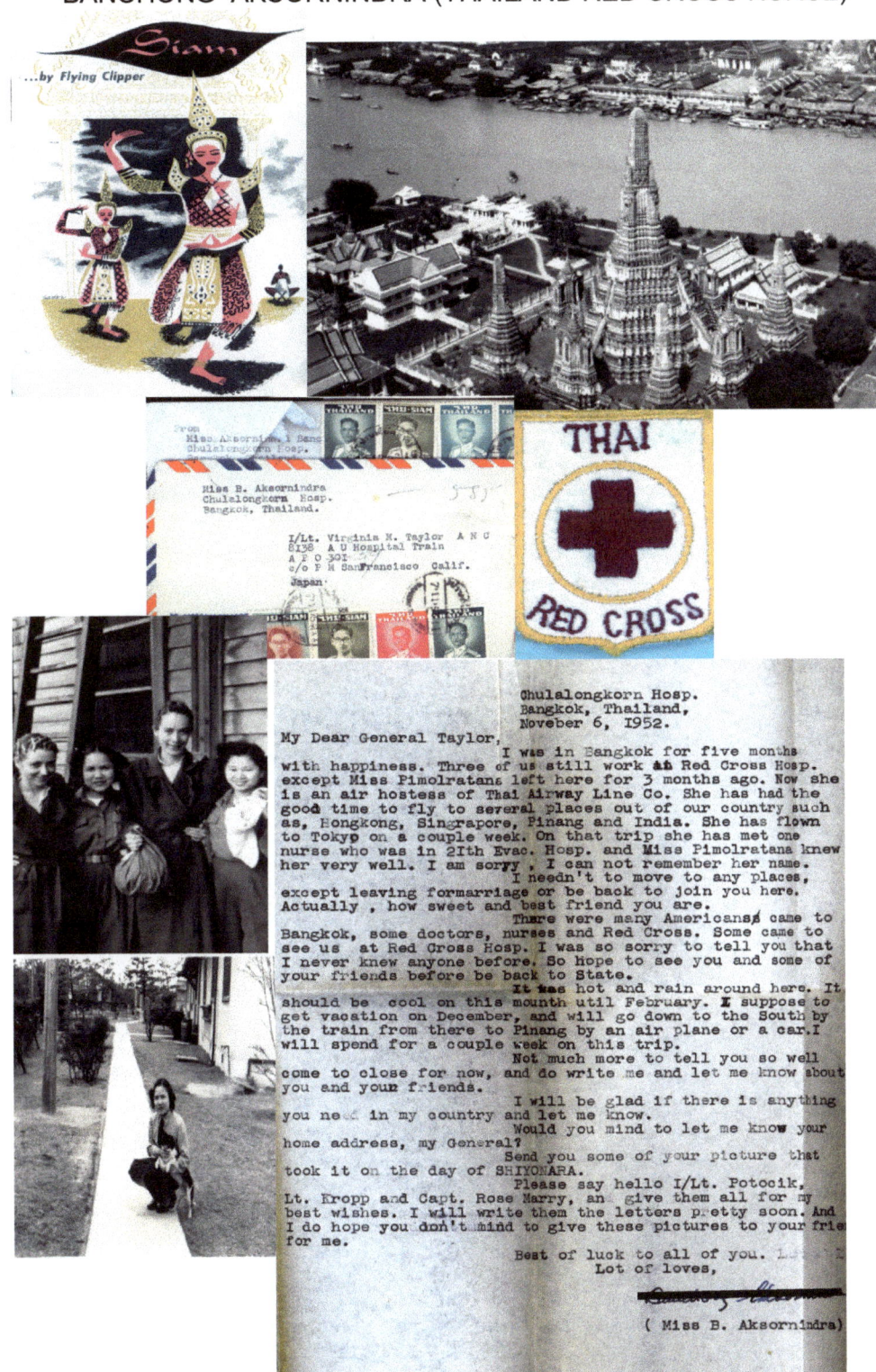

Chulalongkorn Hosp.
Bangkok, Thailand,
Noveber 6, 1952.

My Dear General Taylor,

I was in Bangkok for five months with happiness. Three of us still work at Red Cross Hosp. except Miss Pimolratana left here for 3 months ago. Now she is an air hostess of Thai Airway Line Co. She has had the good time to fly to several places out of our country such as, Hongkong, Singrapore, Pinang and India. She has flown to Tokyo on a couple week. On that trip she has met one nurse who was in 21th Evac. Hosp. and Miss Pimolratana knew her very well. I am sorry, I can not remember her name.

I needn't to move to any places, except leaving for marriage or be back to join you here. Actually, how sweet and best friend you are.

There were many Americans came to Bangkok, some doctors, nurses and Red Cross. Some came to see us at Red Cross Hosp. I was so sorry to tell you that I never knew anyone before. So hope to see you and some of your friends before be back to State.

It was hot and rain around here. It should be cool on this mounth util February. I suppose to get vacation on December, and will go down to the South by the train from there to Pinang by an air plane or a car. I will spend for a couple week on this trip.

Not much more to tell you so well come to close for now, and do write me and let me know about you and your friends.

I will be glad if there is anything you need in my country and let me know.

Would you mind to let me know your home address, my General?

Send you some of your picture that took it on the day of SHIYONARA.

Please say hello I/Lt. Potocik, Lt. Kropp and Capt. Rose Marry, an give them all for my best wishes. I will write them the letters pretty soon. And I do hope you don't mind to give these pictures to your frie for me.

Best of luck to all of you.
Lot of loves,

(Miss B. Aksornindra)

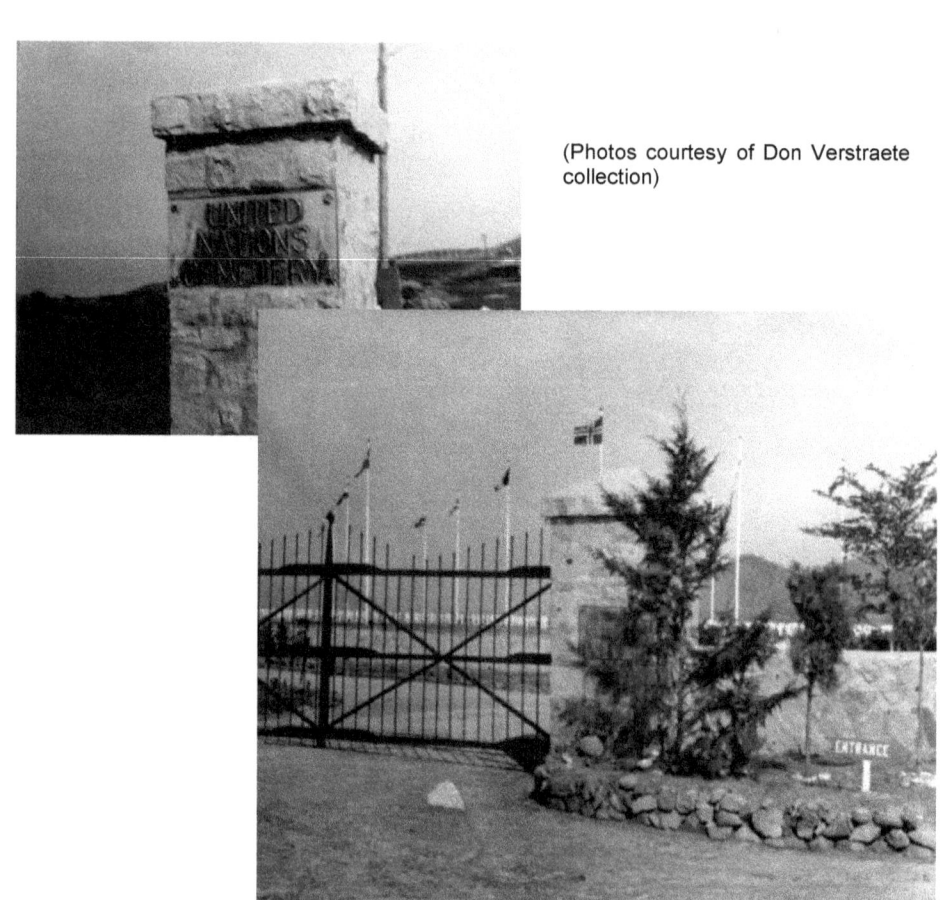

(Photos courtesy of Don Verstraete collection)

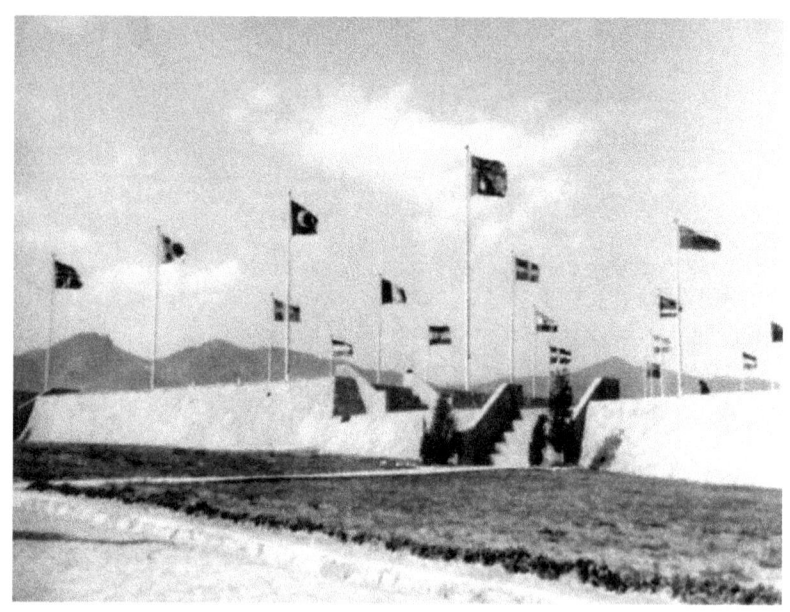

(Photo courtesy of Virginia Taylor collection)

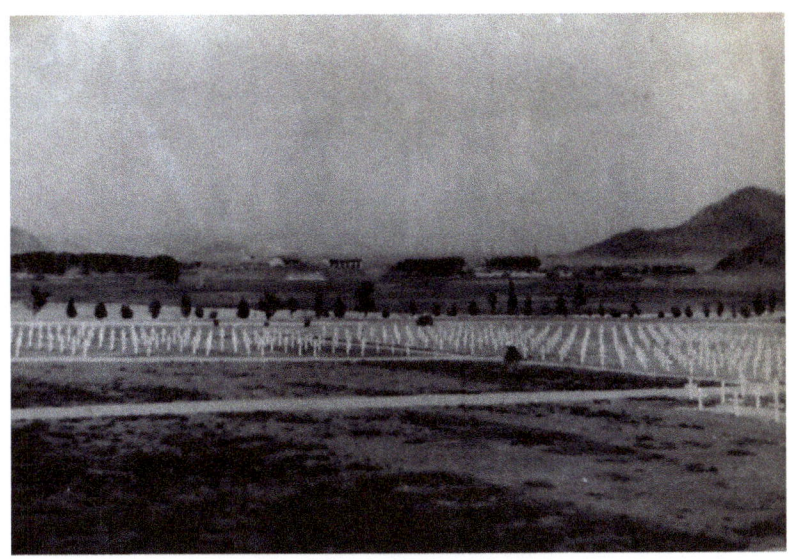

Our Boys Not Coming Home

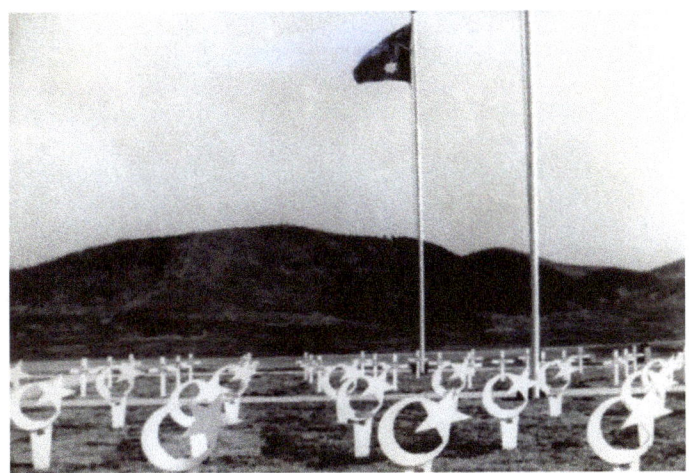

The Turkish soldiers fought bravely too—as did all
who fought for Korea's freedom

(Photos courtesy of Virginia Taylor collection)

DON VERSTRAETE

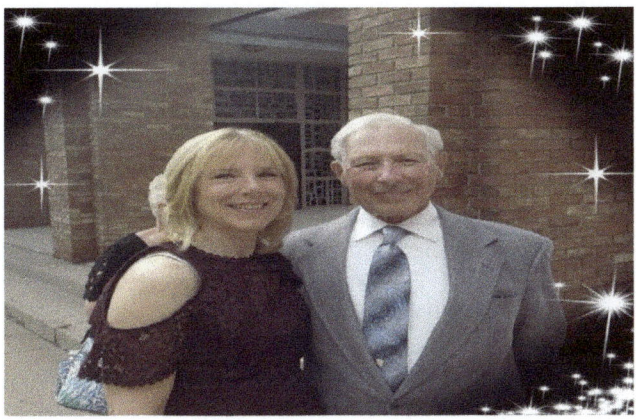

Don with his daughter.

In 1954, Don honorably discharged from the Army and moved back to Detroit, Michigan. Two years later, he married Elizabeth Pierson. The couple had nine children—five boys and four girls—and were married thirty years until her passing in 1986.

From 1957-1963, Don worked for Flag Brothers Shoes in Detroit. First as a salesman, then he was promoted and transferred to Ohio as a manager. Elizabeth missed her family, so Don quit his job and secured a position with Beasley Ford in Detroit. He worked for Beasley for two years until they sold their Ford Dealership, then he hired on with Chrysler in 1966 selling used cars. Within a few months, Chrysler had layoffs and he lost his job. Two months later, he received a call with a better offer from Chrysler to work in their tank plant in Warren, Michigan.

At the Warren facility, he initially worked on the Chrysler Defense Army Project, fork trucks. When the project ended in two years, 1970, he transferred to Chrysler's manufacturing division as a "tank" test driver. From there, he was promoted to the crew manager—quality control inspector of the tanks. Over the years, he worked himself up the ladder, promotions along the way, to General Manager of Quality Control. He worked for Chrysler for twenty-six years until his retirement in 1992 and resided with his mate Karen of thirty years in his Michigan home. Don passed away in April 2022 at the age of 91. He received a copy of this book six months prior and was overjoyed with its publication. "I feared that the history of the 8138th Unit was lost," he had said. "Thank you for remembering us."

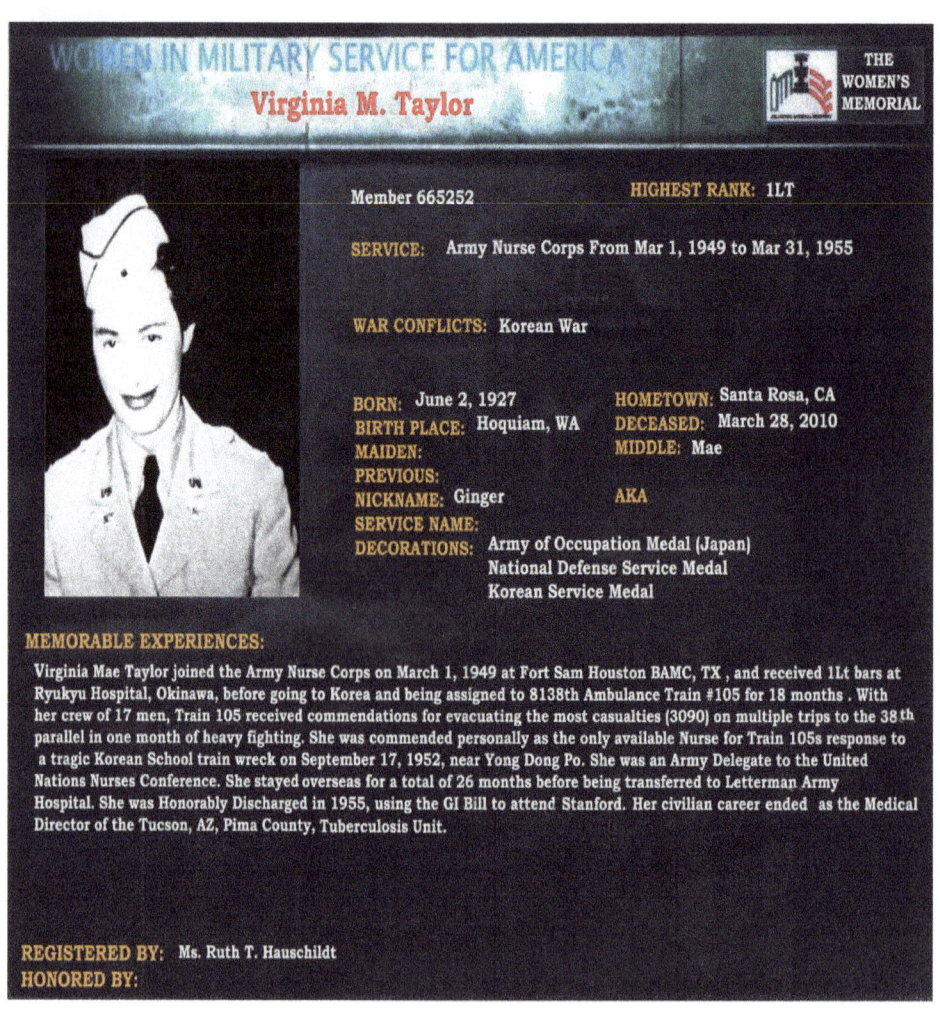

Lt. Virginia Taylor's Women's Memorial database record (Arlington National Cemetery)

The Women's Memorial database at the Arlington National Cemetery has a permanent record of service of Virginia M. Taylor as well as nurses as far back as Florence Nightingale. (www.WomensMemorial.org)

A replica of the hospital trains are at the AMEDD Museum in San Antonio, Texas, where Train 105 Pennsylvania Railroad xylophone dinner chime (pg 72) was donated in 2010.

VIRGINIA TAYLOR

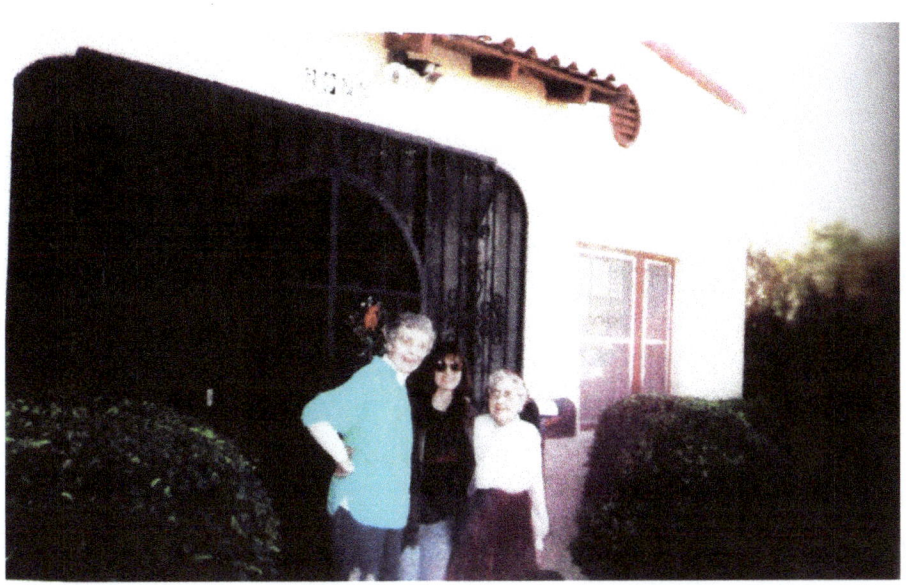

Virginia Taylor with her mother Agnes and
niece KB Taylor (author of this book)
Tucson, AZ 1991

A 1983 letter from Virginia Taylor to Mother Giacomina:

So often I have thought of you and how my life was influenced by you. I still have your letter in my photo album dated July 1945 accepting me to Columbus Hospital School of Nursing. World War II was ending and the Nursing Cadet Corps was also ending. My family was poor and could not pay anything toward my training if the Cadet Corps ended before the September 1945 class. I received a notice from all the hospitals in Seattle asking if my family could pay for my nurses training if the government disbanded the Cadet Nurse Corps. I answered "no" to all the letters including the one received from Columbus Hospital. You were the only one that replied to come to Columbus, and if the Cadet Corps ended, something would be arranged financially. As it turned out, my class was the last of the Cadet Nurse Corps. Such fond memories I have of you, Mother Giacomina, and Mother Delphina, Mother Touboutse, Mother Regina, and my classmates.

In 1944, Virginia's family had moved and left seventeen-year-old Virginia with her boyfriend's family while her boyfriend, Dave, went off to war (WWII). His mother in poor health needed help and both families agreed that Virginia staying behind was the best answer, plus she could graduate with her 1945 Elma (Washington) High School class. When Dave was killed in action, Virginia was devastated. Now without family nearby, Dave gone, and no means for a future, she was at a crossroad. Mother Giacomina offered that helping hand. Virginia graduated from the three-year nursing program at Seattle's Columbus Hospital on full scholarship with straight A's and was the President of her nursing class. In 1949, radio star Kate Smith made an appeal for women to join the U.S. Army Nurses Corps. On March 1, 1949, at Fort Sam Houston, San Antonio, Texas, Virginia's class known as the Kate Smith Cadets, took their oath.

June 1950, Army Corps Nurse Virginia Taylor arrived in Okinawa one week after her twenty-third birthday and several weeks before the start of the Korean War. The next year, she transferred to the hospital trains in Korea.

When Virginia returned to the States, she attended San Francisco State University at night for her Bachelors Degree and worked during the day at Letterman Army Medical Center, San Francisco Presidio to finish her six-year Army obligation.

In 1955, she turned down a promotion as a Captain in the Army, and honorably discharged from service on March 31st the same year. That fall, she attended Stanford University for a Master's Degree on the GI bill. Her thesis was on *The Army Medical Care in Korea*. While attending Stanford, she tutored John Brodie, the football star.

After she received her Master of Science in Public Health Education from Stanford, June 1956, she contacted Mother Giacomina, who was now at the Chicago St. Francis Xavier Cabrini School of Nursing. Virginia applied and was immediately hired at the Hines Teaching Hospital in Illinois as a clinical nursing instructor. The next year, she moved to New Jersey to further her postgraduate training in obstetric nursing and accepted a position on the teaching staff at the Margaret Hague School of Nursing in Jersey City.

Two years of harsh winters sent her west to Nogales, Arizona where she worked four years in the United States Mexican Bracero Program (Mexican temporary worker). In 1962, she moved back to California and worked at the Santa Clara Health Department, taking night classes toward a PhD. She discovered that she preferred "hands on" type of work and accepted a position in Bisbee, AZ working in the United States Bracero Program again. When the program disbanded in 1971, she moved to Tucson and hired on with the Pima County Health Department as the director of tuberculosis programs where she remained until her retirement in 1987.

During her time in Tucson, she sponsored an exchange student from Switzerland for one year, provided scholarships for several children at the Navajo reservation, and built an addition to her home to care for her mother. In her later years, she moved into an independent living apartment and resided there until her passing on March 28, 2010 at the age of 82.

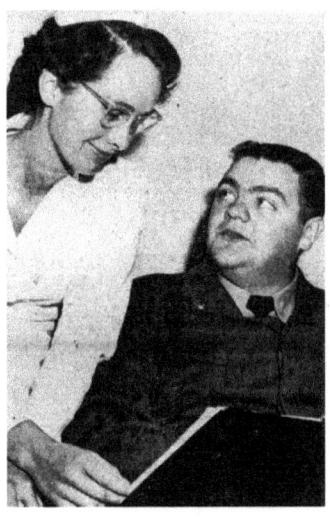

Spanky McFarland of the 1930's Our Gang Comedies with Nurse Virginia Taylor, Letterman Hospital, looking through her Korea scrapbook.

He was recuperating from malaria that he contracted in the Korean War.

This photo with an article later appeared in the newspaper promoting a relief fund for the Korean people.

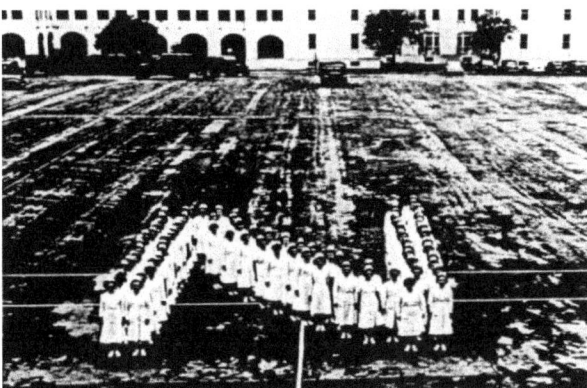

March 1, 1949. Fort Sam Houston, San Antonio, TX. The Kate Smith Cadets. Virginia in far right row, 6th back.

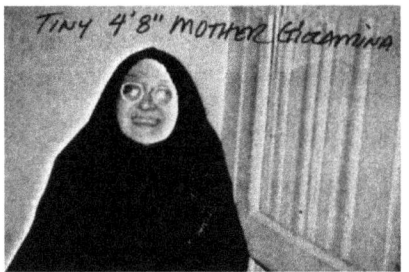

Mother Giacomina
(Photos courtesy of Virginia Taylor collection)

ACKNOWLEDGMENTS

Thank you to my aunt Ruth Taylor Hauschildt for her collaboration with this book. As the family historian and keeper of Virginia's artifacts, her input was invaluable. At age 17, Ruth was the artist of the sketches used for Virginia's 1956 Stanford Thesis.

Thank you to Don Verstraete. His firsthand accounts and photos added to the telling of this story.

Thank you to my husband for his patience for month's on-end of pictures and research spread over our dining-room table.

ABOUT THE AUTHOR

KB Taylor, raised in Grays Harbor County, Washington State, worked as a project-control manager for an aerospace contractor in San Diego. She and her husband now reside in Washington State.

She is an award-winning author whose previous novel is the WILLA award winner *The Seagirls of the Irene*—a children's book based on family history.

WILL ROGERS MEDALLION award winner for *Hattie's Family: Through the Eyes of a Dairymaid* and *Forging Through Unknowns: The Seagirls' Alaska Adventure* (Book 2).

www.kb-taylor.com

NOTES:

[1] American Military History/Korean War/Chapter 25/pg 548
[2] Ibid 1, pg 548
[3] Korean War Educator.org/Participating Nations
[4] National Archives, Revisiting Korea, Exposing Myths of the Forgotten War, Summer 2002, Vol 34, James I. Matray
[5] National Archives, Cold War International History Conference/Paper by William Stueck.
[6] National Archives, Revisiting Korea, Exposing Myths of the Forgotten War, Summer 2002, Vol 34
[7] U.S. Marine Operations in Korea 1950-1953 /The Chosin Reservoir Campaign, Historical Branch, G-3, Headquarters U.S. Marine Corps, Washington D.C/Second Night's Attack on Fox Hill, Pg 190-194
[8] Korean War Educator.org/Participating Nations
[9] Department of Veterans Affairs/American Wars/Nov 2020/Source: DOD Department of Defense
[10] **In theater means** in Korea during the war 1950-1953. <u>Non-theater</u>: those who were stationed in the United States, Germany, and other offsite posts. NOT Korea.
[11] Korean War Educator.org/Participating Nations
[12] The HistoryGuy.com/Korean War Casualties and Statistics; Korean War Educator.org (Civilian lost for both North and South Korea estimated in the millions.)
[13] Map by RMT (Ruth Taylor) 1956
[14] The American Journal of Nursing, *Vol. 52, No. 2/Feb 1952, pg.166-167/Hospital Trains in Korea,* Edith A. Aynes, *R.N, pg 166*
[15] Ibid/Aynes/ Pg 166
[16] Photo released for publication by Army PI Division, March 22, 1956
[17] Cowdrey, *The Medics' War,* Pg 150 Footnote: EUSAK Operations, OSG, 2 Aug 50, sub: Hospital Trains for Far East command, file 322 (Hospital Trains). *The Medics' War*/Center of Military History, United States Army, Washington D.C. 1987/ U.S. Government Printing Office, Washington D.C.(public domain).
[18] Ibid 17, Cowdrey,*Pg 257*
[19] Medical Railroading During the Korean War/Dr. Eric A. Sibul PhD/Railroad History/Fall-Winter 2010/Pg 55-57; V. Taylor letter to parents volunteering for train duty **Aug 1951.** V. Taylor special orders permanently assigning her to **8138 Hospital Train Unit Dec 1951.**
[20] Donald Verstraete, Medic and Car Commander, Train 106, March 1952-May 1953
[21] Ibid 20, Verstraete
[22] The 712th In Korea/Captain Carlton U. Baum/Reading Railroad Magazine/Jan 1953, Vol 17
[23] Transportation Battalion History in the Historical Files of the US Army Transportation Center and School, 712th Battalion
[24] Medical Railroading During the Korean War/Dr. Eric A. Sibul PhD/Railroad History/Fall-Winter 2010/Pg 49-65
[25] Transportation Battalion History in the Historical Files of the US Army Transportation Center and School, 712th, 714th, 765th Battalions
[26] (3d TMRS Runs Busy RR) Pacific Stars and Stripes, Sept 4, 1952,Pg 7. PAO article from Public Information Office (PIO) – public domain by Stars & Stripes, June 12, 2019 e-mail.
[27] (Trans-Medics) Pacific Stars and Stripes, Sept 6, 1952, Pg 6. PAO article from Public Information Office (PIO) – public domain by Stars & Stripes, June 12, 2019.e-mail. Courtesy of Virginia Taylor collection). **Capt. Gerhard J. Newerla—Doctor and Train Commander**
[28] Medical Railroading During the Korean War/Dr. Eric A. Sibul PhD/Railroad History/Fall-Winter 2010/pg 57
[29] Cowdrey,*The Medic's War, pg 257*
[30] Ibid 29, Cowdrey, pg 257
[31] Van Fleet, *Rail Transport and the Winning of Wars*, Pg 33 (Public domain-digitized) https://catalog.hathitrust.org/Record/002020674
[32] Cowdrey,*The Medics' War* ,pg 257
[33] Virginia Taylor's 1956 Stanford Thesis
[34] Back of Photo released for publication by Army PI Division, March 22, 1956 (V. Taylor collection)
[35] Virginia Taylor 1956 Stanford Thesis

[36] Back of Photo released for publication by Army PI Division, March 22, 1956 (V. Taylor collection)

[37] Back of Photo released for publication by Army PI Division, March 22, 1956 (V. Taylor collection)

[38] Train #106 (Don Verstraete) only transported South Korean soldiers. One of his routes was to the 171st Evacuation Hospital in Taejon, which cared for the Korean Service Corps alone. Cowdrey, the Medics's War, pg 329.

[39] Back of Photo released for publication by Army PI Division, March 22, 1956 (V. Taylor collection)

[40] Cowdrey, The Medics' War, Pg145; Don Verstraete Pg 45 firsthand knowledge.

[41] Ibid 40, Pg 186

[42] Train #106 (Don Verstraete) only transported South Korean soldiers.

[43] (*International Angles of Mercy*) Pacific Stars & Stripes, February 2, 1952, Public Information Office (PIO), Public Domain per Stars & Stripes June 12, 2019 e-mail. .

[44] Mossman, Billy (1990), Ebb and Flow, Vol 5, US Army in Korean War. Gov Printing Office p. 493; History Army Military/Books/Korea/Truce/Chapter 5 (The New War); Korean War Campaigns UN Summer-Fall Offensive (July-Nov 1951).

[45] American Military History/Korean War

[46] Cowdrey, *The Medics' War*, Pg 75

[47] . Transportation Battalion History in the Historical Files of the US Army Transportation Center and School, 712th, pg 10

[48] Cowdrey, *The Medics' War*, Pg 117-118

[49] The Xylophone was donated to the AMEDD Museum, San Antonio, Texas by Virginia's sister Ruth
in 2010

[50] Cowdrey,*The Medics' War*, pg 200

[51] Cowdrey, *the Medics' War*, pg 232

[52] (*Hospital Train Sets Frontline Record*, 1952.) PAO article from Public Information Office (PIO) – public domain.

[53] (*Twisted Cars Clog Bridge*), Pacific Stars & Stripes, Sept 17, 1952, Pgs 1 & 16, Bill FizGerald. Permission to publish from Stars & Stripes June 12,2019 e-mail.

[54] Transportation Battalion History in the Historical Files of the US Army Transportation Center and School, 712th, pg 10

[55] (*A Wounded Man Comes Back*) December 06, 1952, Pages 8-9. Photographer: Ken Patterson. Permission to publish received from Stars & Stripes, June 12, 2019 e-mail (News article courtesy of Virginia Taylor collection.)

[56] Historyguy.com/Korean War Casualties and Statistics

[57] Courtesy of National Archives, Signal Corps

[58] Signal Corps III, ADC 8665, Army Pictorial Center (Public domain)

[59] Goulden, *Korea: The Untold Story of the War*, pp 548-650

[60] Cowdrey, *The Medics Wa*r, PP 345-350. **(Updated numbers from Koreawar.org/history: Communist repatriated 684 U.N. sick and wounded. The U.N. returned 1,030 Chinese and 5,194 Koreans.)**

[61] Cowdrey,*The Medics War*, P 350

REFERENCE DETAIL:

C.G. <@ stripes.com>
Cc: Permission <Permission@stripes.com>
I took a look at all the scan you sent. Some of them are not ours so we do not own the rights to those and cannot grant permission, others are in public domain, so you do not need permission, and a few are ours. I'd be more than happy to grant you permission to republish the ones that are ours in your book.

Details for each of the articles/images are noted below. I noted the date of publication for each of the articles/images below when I looked them up so you can include those in your book.

PAO articles:
Several of the articles appear to be from the Public Information Office (PIO), recognizable by the "WITH THE (UNIT DESIGNATION) –in the dateline." These can be considered to be in the Public Domain.
"3rd TMRS Runs Busy Railroad," published in Pacific Stars and Stripes Sept. 4, 1952. Page 7
"Trans-Medics," published in Pacific Stars and Stripes Sept. 6, 1952, page 6
"Angels of Mercy," Pacific Stars and Stripes, February 2, 1952, pages 6 and 7

Stars and Stripes articles/photos:
"A Wounded Man Comes Back," published December 06, 1952, Pages 8-9. Photographer: Ken Patterson
"Twisted Cars Clog Bridge," Pacific Stars and Stripes, September 17,1952, pages 1 and 16. Reporter: Bill FitzGerald
Stars and Stripes War Map - Unfortunately, I was unable to locate this map in our historic newspaper archive - it's often hard to find illustrations as the text in it is often not recognized as such by the search engine, **but I will include it in the agreement.**

C. G.
Supervisory Archivist & Licensing and Permissions Representative
@stripes.com
www.stripes.com

---

2. Albert E. Cowdrey worked for the U.S. Army Center of Military History. *The Medics' War* was written while he was chief of the Medical History Branch at the Center of Military History. (Note: work created by a federal government employee or officer is in public domain.)

---

3. Many digitized images by the Signal Corps can be viewed through the National Archives Catalog. Because the photographs were taken by military personnel while on duty they **are considered** to be in the **public domain**. Nov 22, 2019

---

4. Korean War Project (Koreanwar.org/Ted Barker) permission to use quotations on Author's Note.

www.ingramcontent.com/pod-product-compliance
Lightning Source LLC
Chambersburg PA
CBHW040042100526
44583CB00027BA/3255